28 Days TO CLEAN

Ryan Chapman
with recipes by Heidi Boortz

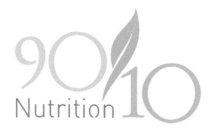

90/10 Nutrition

28 Days To Clean by Ryan Chapman
Published by BASE Training LLC

9010nutrition.com
28daystoclean.com

Cover and interior design by Ryan Chapman
Recipes by Ryan Chapman and Heidi Boortz
Photo Credits: Carrie Patterson/pg. 6, Heidi Boortz/pg. 170. All other photographs by Ryan Chapman

ISBN: 978-1-945137-21-1
10 9 8 7 6 5 4 3 2 1
First Edition

I'd like to thank the following people for helping to make this book a reality:

Heidi Boortz - You are a genius with your recipes. Thank you so much for all of the recipes you have created for 90/10 Nutrition, many of which are in this book in some form.

The 28 Days To Clean Test Group - Thank you to the 20+ people who went through this program diligently in a messy Word document format and gave me detailed feedback.

Jamie Swift - Thank you so much for going through this program several times, giving me advice and feedback, encouraging me, and even helping me edit this book. You are a dear friend.

My Family - Thank you so much to my wife, kids, and other close family members for putting up with late night work, helping me edit, and being an encouragement to me throughout this process.

The 90/10 Members - Finally, I want to thank my 90/10 Nutrition family. I appreciate your support through this project and throughout the last 7 years building 90/10 Nutrition into the program that it is today.

CONTENTS

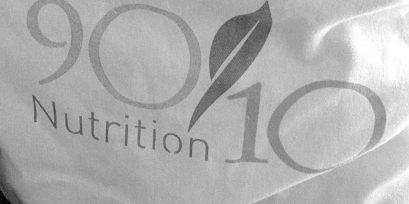
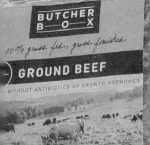

INTRODUCTION

In early 2004, I sat in a small airport in Kalispell, MT with my Dad. I was 23 years old, just 6 months out of college as an engineer, and as out of shape as I had ever been. There are very few pictures of me during this time. The picture on the right was taken 6 months earlier when I graduated from college and was probably a good 15 pounds lighter than I was that day in the airport.

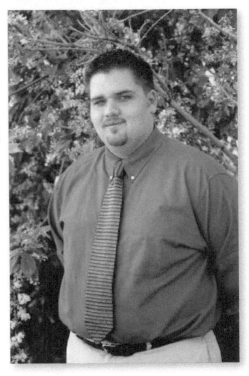

I could tell my Dad had wanted to say something about my weight all weekend during our vacation at Big Mountain in Whitefish, MT, and he eventually did there in the airport. He simply said, almost out of the blue, "You gotta do something, bud." I didn't need an explanation for the otherwise random comment. I knew exactly what he meant.

Now, we could either spend the rest of this book analyzing the mental effects of that comment and the rest of my childhood, or we could talk about what happened after that and how it led to writing this book. I'm guessing that you're not here for a detailed account of my childhood emotional baggage, so I'll save that for another time.

That day, my Dad and I committed to sending daily emails with a food journal to keep each other accountable. This wasn't new territory for me though. I weighed around 275 pounds at that point, but dieting was certainly not foreign to me. Like many overweight people, I'd been dieting most of my life. I can still vividly remember going to Taco Bell as a kid and asking for the nutritional information pamphlet so I could count my calories. I lost 35 or 40 pounds on a 1200 calorie diet when I was 12 years old.

By the time I left for college, I had done 1200 calorie diets, 1500 calorie diets,

Jenny Craig, Slim Fast, and the cabbage soup diet (the one they would use for heart surgery patients that need to lose weight). On all of them, I would lose weight while I was on it, but I never actually changed my eating habits. As soon as I would stop the diet, the weight would come back. Often, it would be more than the original weight I had lost on the diet.

Despite all of that, I went back to my gold standard 1500 calorie diet for my accountability plan with my Dad. Sure, I would eat salads and other stuff I thought was good for me, but the main goal was always keeping under 1500 calories. Diet soda was a 60+ ounce per day habit and I would often skip meals or eat very small amounts so I could have enough calories left for ice cream.

The first few weeks on the new (err...uh...same old) plan were business as usual. I lost weight like I always did on a 1500 calorie diet and I started hating the restriction of it all around week 2. I was hungry, feeling deprived, and craving all the things I couldn't have.

Fortunately, this time didn't end the way other diet attempts had in the past. Two things happened during the first few weeks of that diet that I believe were critical to my health journey. First, I met my future wife in the first week after starting the diet. Secondly, some buddies from work heard I was on a diet and decided to make it a contest. Those two factors pushed me to stick with my plan for much longer than I ever had. My Dad and I stopped emailing around 6 weeks in, but I didn't stop dieting. In fact, later in the weight loss contest, we decided to do a sprint triathlon at the end and that pushed me even more.

By May of 2005, I was down 80 pounds from that day in the airport and was about to get married. I was also the narrowly defeated silver medalist of the weight loss contest and about to complete my first triathlon.

I wish I could tell you that the entire year I spent on a 1500 calorie diet ended up being no big deal, but I can't. That year was incredibly difficult. The support of the contest and my future wife along with the motivation to look good at my wedding and complete my first triathlon without dying was enough to carry me through, but all the typical things that everyone hates about dieting were right there the whole time. It was tough.

It's possible that you haven't personally stayed on a diet for a year and lost 80 lbs. It's possible that you haven't completed any triathlons either. But, there's a good chance the first part of my story isn't much different than your story.

I can't count the number of times I've heard versions of my story in other people's lives. I've met so many people who have been on that same "diet rollercoaster" that I was on for 20 years. Many of them have been on it for even longer. They've tried all the diets. Atkin's, keto, South Beach, low fat, low carb, high fat, raw vegan, Slim Fast, and maybe even the heart surgery cabbage soup diet.

If that's you, then you're definitely in the right place, because what happened *after* I lost all that weight is what really changed my life. It's what led me to create the 90/10 Nutrition system (more on that later) and write this book.

I'm going to share that story with you in the next few pages. Don't skip reading the first part of this book so you can get to the "plan". I know it can be tempting to say, "just show me what to do. I don't care about the why." But, from someone just like you, please trust me when I say that you won't regret taking a little time to read what I'm about to share with you.

I'm excited to guide you through the next 4 weeks, so turn the page and let's get started.

Thank you,

Ryan Chapman
90/10 Nutrition

PART I
CLEAN EATING

ABOUT CLEAN EATING

If you read the introduction to this book and related, you might also be wondering how this is possible for so many people. How did we get here? Is it normal and unpreventable for people to be suffering through counting calories and hating dieting? Is this just how dieting is supposed to be? I certainly used to think so. I used to think hunger and deprivation were just normal parts of dieting, and I viewed dieting this way as a necessary evil of life.

I suppose you can probably guess that I no longer view eating this way, and I want to do my very best to make sure that you don't either. So, in the first part of this book, I am just going to give a brief look at the line of thinking that changed my mind and led me to "clean eating".

DEFINING CLEAN EATING

First of all, let's define clean eating. You may find different definitions around the internet and in different books. The term "clean eating" isn't regulated in any way that I know of, so there is no definitive set of rules to help define it.

While there does seem to be a general consensus around the term in many circles, it can vary at least a bit. I originally hesitated to use the term at all when I first started talking about this way of eating. In fact, my first blog on this topic back in 2010 was titled "The Low Ingredient Diet". I'll talk more about that in a minute, but I ended up associating with "clean eating" because there was a thriving community around it and it seemed to capture the overall concept better than "low ingredient".

Here's how I define Clean Eating:

"Eat foods in a state as close to their natural state as possible. Minimize or avoid refined grains, refined sugars, overly-processed foods and artificial ingredients."

In short, clean eating is about just eating real food. For this reason, clean eating doesn't focus as much

> **ℹ REMINDER**
>
> This section is for your understanding only. The 28-day plan in this book is completely laid out for you. You won't need to make a bunch of decisions in order to complete the plan. However, I think this understanding will help you a lot and set you up for continued success after the program, so don't skip this section.

on macronutrient values such as carbohydrate grams, fat grams, protein grams, and calories. Food is evaluated based on the ingredients list rather than the macronutrients (or "macros").

With clean eating, you tend to shop around the perimeter of the grocery store where you find foods with only one ingredient like "carrots" and "salmon". If you purchase packaged foods with an ingredients label, you read the ingredients and watch for anything that isn't something you recognize as real food.

or not. Sometimes it's a confusing blend of all of them and sometimes it focuses on just one of them.

Maybe you've heard someone say something like, "It's simple really. Burn more calories than you consume." Or, maybe you've heard one of the various debates focused on one macronutrient such as fat or carbohydrates (protein usually gets a pass or even a gold star in this debate).

For most of the last 4 or 5 decades, fat was the overwhelming black sheep of the bunch. Dietary fat intake

> **Eat foods in a state as close to their natural state as possible. Minimize or avoid refined grains, refined sugars, overly-processed foods and artificial ingredients.**

In most cases, foods and food groups such as grains and dairy are not completely cut out of clean eating programs.

WHY CLEAN EATING?

For years, the prevailing conventional wisdom has had us looking at some combination of macronutrients to determine if a food is healthy to eat

took the blame for obesity and heart disease starting in the '50s or '60s and became the absolute enemy by the late '70s.

More recently, fat has found redemption while carbohydrates have become the enemy. It seems everywhere you look someone is trying to limit or even completely eliminate carbs from their diet.

How is it that we don't know which macronutrients are the bad ones and which ones are the good ones? Well, maybe it's because none of them are bad! Maybe it's because we have created our own confusion.

How We Got Here

Go with me in your mind for just a second and imagine a time when there were no grocery stores, no packaging, no food processing plants, no tractors or even fields full of crops, no animal agriculture, and no centralized or industrialized food production of any kind. Just imagine the time. It existed at some point in the past. At some point, we had to hunt and gather our food from the wild.

When food was something that had to be hunted and gathered, you can imagine it was more about how to get *enough* food to survive than it was about how to make sure you don't eat *too much* and gain weight. There most likely was little to no concern about the fat content, carbohydrate content or protein content of the foods. In fact, many of the foods that we have avoided at the behest of the USDA for last 50 years would have been very highly prized for their calorie density (high fat foods). Of course, this wouldn't have been talked about in terms of fat grams but it would have been understood through experiencing how those foods helped you last longer between meals.

Fast forward to today and you see that we are almost completely disconnected from the source of our food. Between us (the consumers of the food) and the source, lies food distributors, food manufacturers, and farmers (at a minimum).

Many of the foods in the stores do not resemble anything close to a food you could find in nature or even on the farm. They've been processed to be sweeter, or to have less fat, or to stay fresh on the shelf longer, or to be more convenient to grab on the go (or all of those).

This is a very new development and it seems to correlate very closely with the rise in obesity and disease over the last 100 years or so. Although we have tried to pin those issues on one ingredient or the other, one macronutrient or the other, or one food group or the other, the main thing that has changed during that time is that the food itself is no longer just real, whole food.

I'm not suggesting that we go back to hunting and gathering our food from the wild. That seems pretty unrealistic and even unnecessary.

However, we can make a move toward real food even within the current food system that we have, and that's exactly what clean eating is all about.

Ingredients Matter

As I mentioned in the introduction, I used calorie counting to lose weight back in 2005. Lunches for me would often be a microwaveable lunch from the freezer at work. Snacks might be something like 100 calorie packs of little cookies or Peanut M&M's. I would drink diet sodas and use snack bars touting high protein and using artificial sweeteners. I would often eat less during the day so I could save calories for ice cream at night.

Then, one day, someone told me to try counting *ingredients* instead of *calories*. Of course, this idea didn't make much sense to me at first, but when I saw the difference in the ingredients between real food and processed "diet food", it started to come together.

Let me give you the exact example that opened my ideas to the power of ingredients and real food back in 2010.

Let's imagine a typical start to the day for someone on a calorie restriction diet (this was literally me):

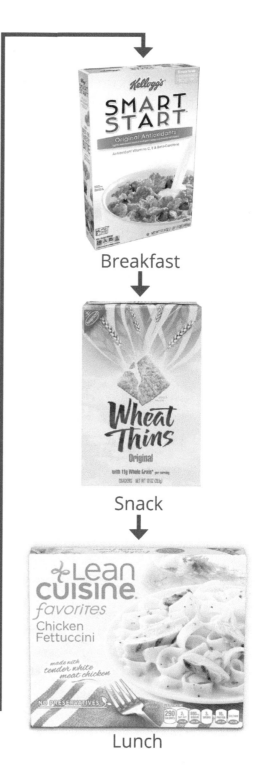

Breakfast

Snack

Lunch

Now, to me, that used to seem like a great start. Each of those items have some healthy buzzwords on the box (lean, smart, heart healthy, whole grains) and they are relatively low in calories.

Let's just take a look at the ingredients of those three items.

This is exactly what made me decide to give this "clean eating" thing a try. Look at the list of ingredients below!

The first paragraph is the cereal, the second is the Wheat Thins crackers, and the third is a Chicken Fettucine Alfredo Lean Cuisine.

There are over 100 ingredients in those three items with brackets upon brackets of additives!

Cereal Ingredients: Rice, whole grain wheat, sugar, whole grain oats, brown sugar syrup, contains 2% or less of rice flour, corn syrup, salt, malt flavor, honey, barley malt extract, cinnamon, natural flavor, mixed tocopherols (vitamin E) for freshness. Vitamins and Minerals: Vitamin C (ascorbic acid), reduced iron, vitamin E acetate, niacinamide, vitamin B6 (pyridoxine hydrochloride), vitamin B1 (thiamin hydrochloride), folic acid, vitamin B2 (riboflavin), beta-carotene, vitamin D3, vitamin B12. (smartlabel.kelloggs.com)

Wheat Thins (Original) Ingredients: Whole Grain Wheat Flour, Unbleached Enriched Flour (Wheat Flour, Niacin, Reduced Iron, Thiamine Mononitrate {Vitamin B1}, Riboflavin {Vitamin B2}, Folic Acid), Soybean Oil, Sugar, Cornstarch, Malt Syrup (from Barley and Corn), Salt, Invert Sugar, Monoglycerides, Leavening (Calcium Phosphate and/or Baking Soda), Vegetable Color (Annatto Extract, Turmeric Oleoresin). (walmart.com)

Lean Cuisine Ingredients: blanched fettuccini (water, semolina, wheat gluten), skim milk, cooked chicken tenderloin (chicken tenderloins, water, seasoning (modified corn starch, sugar, potassium chloride, yeast extract, dextrose, spice, onion powder, garlic powder, paprika), soybean oil, isolated soy protein, salt, sodium phosphates), broccoli, water, 2% or less of cream, modified cornstarch, salt, enzyme modified parmesan cheese paste (parmesan cheese (cultured part-skim milk, salt, enzymes), water, whey protein concentrate (from milk), reduced fat milk, milk protein concentrate, enzymes, nonfat milk, cultures), parmesan cheese paste (granular and parmesan cheese (pasteurized milk, cheese cultures, salt, enzymes), water, salt, lactic acid, citric acid), soybean oil, bleached wheat flour, romano cheese product ((pasteurized cow's milk, cheese cultures, salt, enzymes), water, salt, lactic acid), butterfat, whey protein concentrate, cheese flavor (cheddar cheese (cultured milk, salt, enzymes), water, salt, enzymes, cultures, phosphoric acid, xanthan gum), spices, mono-&diglycerides, xanthan gum, flavor (maltodextrin, flavoring and modified food starch), yeast extract, seasoning (wheat starch, extracts of annatto and turmeric color, natural flavor). (leancuisine.com)

Now, watch what happens when we create meals and snacks from whole foods.

Here is an example:

- **Replace the cereal with some rolled oats sweetened with honey**

- **Replace the Wheat Thins with some fruit (such as blueberries)**

- **Replace the Lean Cuisine with Chicken, Brown Rice, Green Beans, and real Butter**

In this example, we have breakfast, a snack, and lunch with only 7 ingredients! Of course, you might add some milk or almond milk to the oats, you might add some spices to the chicken, you may salt the green beans, etc. You still won't come anywhere near 138 ingredients and you'll be able to pronounce them all.

I was able to pick items that come out to almost the exact same macronutrients counts (calories, carbs, fat, and protein) as the processed meal, but with only a fraction of the ingredients. I actually plugged both meals into a tracking app to show how similar they are in total macronutrients.

Now, which of these two options do you think your body will appreciate, recognize, and utilize more efficiently?

This is the question that made me try low ingredient eating and eventually fall in love with the clean eating philosophy.

	Processed Food	Real Food
Total Calories	610	614
Fat (g)	11	9
Protein (g)	22	21
Carbohydrates (g)	109	115
Number of Ingredients	~130	<10

HOW TO EAT CLEAN

As I mentioned earlier and as you can see from the examples, reading ingredients is the cornerstone of clean eating. It's about **real food** ingredients that your body was designed to consume. It's not about eliminating food groups, it's about eliminating **fake food**! This means that we can't rely on certain parts of the nutrition label to tell the real story about our food.

Since we are more concerned with what ingredients are in our food (and where they come from) than we are about the calories, protein, carbs, and fat, we have to look at the ingredients list on the packaging rather than the nutrition facts section of the label.

The ideal situation would be to buy mostly things that don't have packaging, such as fruits, veggies, meats from the butcher, raw nuts and seeds, etc. However, the truth of the matter is that you will likely buy things that come in a package, so you need to know how to find the good ones.

Starting in the next section, I'm going to give you the 90/10 "traffic light" system for clean eating. The red, yellow, and green system makes it super easy to choose clean foods just about anywhere. But, before I do that, I think it is helpful to give some basic rules of thumb for clean eating even if you aren't using the system I developed. Of course, I'm partial to my system, but you don't have to use my brand in order to eat clean.

So, on the facing page are some guiding principles you can use to choose clean eating foods.

Remember, if you follow the plan for the next 28 days, everything is basically done for you. Don't get too hung up on any of this information.

Just think about these things as you go through the plan and go to the grocery store over the next 4 weeks.

ⓘ NOTE

You can find helpful additional resources such as printables and links online at www.28daystoclean.com/resources (or simply use the QR code to the right).

BASIC RULES FOR CLEAN EATING

• **_Don't eat anything your great grandmother wouldn't recognize as food_** - This really only applies if you're reading this near the time that I'm writing this. To be safe, let's just say that you shouldn't eat anything that someone born before about 1900 wouldn't recognize as food. High fructose corn syrup (a corn-based sweetener you'll find in many processed junk foods), for example, was invented in the 1950s. Anyone born around 1900 wouldn't have had much access to hydrogentated fats (trans fats) either. Thinking in terms of what someone had available as foods up until somewhere around the early 1900s can be helpful in choosing real foods

• **_Don't eat ingredients you couldn't easily buy somewhere else in the store_** - If you can't walk to another aisle in the store and easily buy the ingredients in the packaged food you're holding, put it back on the shelf and don't buy it. Take the Lean Cuisine on page 4 as an example. Could you purchase maltodextrin by itself in the store? Possibly, but it's not something you would be likely to see in a recipe you would cook at home. Could you buy modified food starch or modified corn starch by themselves to use in recipes? Probably not, but you can find these things in a great many processed food products. If you wouldn't buy it and put it in a home cooked recipe, don't buy a product that has it in the ingredients either.

• **_Don't eat it if you can't pronounce it_** - There are maybe a few exceptions to this rule. Quinoa would be one of them (it's "keen-wah", by the way), but that's not the kind of thing this rule is about. Hopefully you understand that this rule doesn't mean that you can eat it if you learn how to pronounce it by consulting a dictionary. This rule is really just another way of saying what the first two rules say as well. Don't eat food products, eat real foods. If you see chemical-sounding names that you don't recognize like polydextrose, maltodextrin, and mono- and diglycerides, it's most likely a processed food that isn't a good clean eating choice.

THE 90/10 SYSTEM

90/10 Nutrition takes the simple rules laid out on the last page and makes them into an easy-to-follow system. This is the system I used to create this 28-day plan.

You will only need the the 90/10 system during the next 4 weeks if you decide to make a substitution on a recipe and you want to stay within the guidelines.

Otherwise, you won't need it until you transition to your own plan at the end of the 4 weeks, and that will be covered in detail in the transition section so you are ready to go when the time comes.

In the transition section, starting on page 89, I list all of the resources we have for learning to do the 90/10 system. So, I won't go into extreme detail here.

The system is based on three simple food lists known as the green tier, the yellow tier, and the red tier. It's like a traffic light. Green means "go", yellow means "caution", red means "stop".

On the next few pages, you'll find the actual tiers. To use them, you simply compare the ingredients in foods to the tiers. You can find just about any ingredient on the tiers.

So, whether you're buying fresh foods from the farmer's market or packaged foods from the center aisles at the grocery store, you can use the tiers to guide you.

Now, here are the rules for using the 90/10 tiers (which can be seen on the pages that follow):

USING THE 90/10 TIERS

- **Eat 90% (or more) of your food from the** Green Tier - The green tier is the good stuff. This is where you'll find fruits, vegetables, meats, whole grains, nuts, and healthy fats. You'll also find sweet potatoes, plain yogurt, and more.

- **Eat 10% (or less) of your food from the** Yellow Tier - This tier has the "compromise" foods on it. You'll find natural sweeteners like honey and maple syrup on this tier. You'll also find beer and wine, white rice, white bread, and white potatoes on the yellow tier.

- **Eat 0% from the Red Tier** - This is where you'll find processed sugar, artificial sweeteners, and all the highly processed junk foods. This is the stuff you'll need to stay away from when eating clean. Of course, when we say "0%", we're referring to your daily diet. If you have a planned special occasion that involves red tier items, that's pretty normal.

THE GREEN TIER

PRIMARY VEGGIES
Artichokes
Asparagus
Beets
Bok Choy
Broccoli
Brussels Sprouts
Cabbage
Carrots
Cauliflower
Celery
Cucumbers
Eggplant
Greens, Leafy (all types)
Green Beans
Jicama
Lettuce
Mushrooms
Okra
Onions
Peppers (bell and sweet)
Radishes
Sprouts
Squash
Tomatoes
Zucchini

OTHER FOODS
Lemon and Lime Juice
Vinegars
Mustard
Herbs (fresh and dry)
Spices
Garlic
Ginger
Flavor Extracts
Black Coffee (unsweetened)
Tea (unsweetened)
Broths (low sodium, no sugar)
Stevia
Water

LEAN PROTEINS
Beef, Lean (<10% fat)
Buffalo, Lean (<10% fat)
Chicken (all)
Cottage Cheese (Any Fat %)
Eggs
Dairy Milk
Fish (preferrably wild caught)
Greek or Regular Yogurt, Plain
Pork Tenderloin and Chops
Protein Powder (unsweetened)
Shellfish
Soy Milk (unsweetened)
Tempeh
Tofu
Turkey and other fowl (all)
Veal
Wild Game, Lean (<10% fat)

SECONDARY VEGGIES AND GRAINS
Beans (low sodium if canned)
Bread (100% whole grain, no HFCS)
Corn
Cous Cous (100% whole grain)
Edamame
Grains, Whole
Lentils
Oats (rolled or steel cut)
Pasta (100% whole grain)
Peas
Purple Potatoes
Quinoa
Rice (Brown and Wild)
Brown Rice Milk (unsweetened)
Spelt
Sweet Potato/Yams

HEALTHY FATS
Almond Milk (unsweetened)
Avocado
Butter
Cheeses, Various
Coconut (unsweetened)
Coconut Milk (unsweetened)
Coconut Oil
Flaxseed
Nuts
Nut Butters
Olives
Olive Oil
Seeds
Seed Butters

FRUIT
Apples
Apricots
Banana
Berries
Cherries
Citrus Fruits
Dates
Figs
Grapes
Kiwi
Mango
Melons
Peaches/Nectarines
Papaya
Pears
Pineapples
Plantains
Plums/prunes
Raisins

THE YELLOW TIER

PROTEINS
Bacon (uncured is best)
Beef, Lean (>10% fat)
Buffalo or Wild Game, Lean (>10% fat)
Canadian Bacon
Ham
Lamb
Pork (fatty cuts)

CARBOHYDRATES
Agave Nectar
Alcohol (hard liquor)
Beer
Bread/Bagel products (if not 100% whole grain)
Tortilla Chips or Fried Tortillas
Crackers (not 100% whole grain)
Honey
Juice (from concentrate)
Maple Syrup (pure)
Molasses
Pasta (not 100% whole grain)
Potatoes (white, not fried)
Rice (white)
Soy Sauce
Tortillas (flour, not 100% whole grain)
Wine

FATS
Canola and Vegetable Oils
Cream
Half and Half

THE RED TIER

Artificial Sweeteners (sucralose, aspartame, saccharine, etc)
Fillers, Preservatives, chemicals you don't recognize as food
Fried Foods (excludes lightly sauteeing in Green Tier oils)
High Fructose Corn Syrup
Processed meats (cured with chemicals and preservatives and sugar)
Hydrogenated Foods
Maltodextrin
Margarine
Sports Drinks and Sports Nutrition Products (unless using properly for training)
Sugar
Sugar Alcohols (anything ending in -tol)

PART II
THE PLAN

ABOUT THIS PLAN

The plan that follows is your 28-day plan for clean eating. The next few pages will outline important notes, how to shop and source food, guidelines for substitution, hydration, relaxation and sleep, exercise recommendations, transitioning at the end, and more. You'll also find a page dedicated to each day of this 28-day plan. The daily plan pages will tell you exactly what to eat for each meal and snack along with helpful tips and thoughts for the day. You'll also see a summary calendar view and a shopping list at the beginning of each week.

IMPORTANT NOTES

• This plan is set up to outline every meal and snack for 1 person. All quantities in the recipes are intended to reflect the amount needed for 1 person. If you are doing this plan with your significant other or a family, you will need to modify amounts accordingly.

• This plan is gluten free in that it does not call for any ingredients that contain gluten. However, if you know you have a sensitivity or allergy, you need to read allergen labels since I cannot guarantee there wouldn't be manufacturer cross-contamination. This plan is simply intended to call out ingredients that do not contain any gluten. It is not "certified gluten free".

• This plan uses some dairy in cultured form (Greek yogurt) and butter or ghee. It does not use cheese, milk, or other forms of dairy. You can easily substitute the yogurt recipes for some of the other recipes in the plan (per the instructions for substitutions that follow) if you desire to be completely dairy free.

• There are many tasty breakfast, lunch, snack, and dinner recipes in this plan, but the plan does repeat recipes. You won't find a different recipe every single day for breakfast, lunch or snacks. I could have done 28 different recipes for each course, but I don't believe that is realistic for most people. If you're anything like me, you're perfectly fine eating the same thing for breakfast and lunch a few times a week (if not more often than that). Also, I want your shopping to be as efficient as possible. If you have some repeats each week and use the same ingredients in different meals, your shopping will be easier.

SUBSTITUTING MEALS

The fact that this program details every meal on every single day does not mean that you can't make substitutions. It is simply set up this way so you can easily plug yourself into the program without having to do much meal planning on your own. However, I realize that some people have special schedules, allergies, tastes, and preferences. So, I've set up some guidelines if you wish to change the meal plan around a bit during the course of this 28-day program. It's up to you if you use the guidelines below to personalize your 28 days or take them on as is.

GUIDELINES FOR SUBSTITUTING MEALS

• You can substitute any breakfast for any other breakfast in the plan provided you meet the rest of the requirements below.

• You can substitute ingredients in recipes as long as they are on the same tier or higher (see pages 19 - 20 for tiers) and they meet the rest of the requirements below. Example: You should not substitute white rice for brown rice because white rice is on the yellow tier and brown rice is on the green tier. However, you may substitute cauliflower rice for brown rice because both would be green tier.

• Make sure you maintain lots of variety. It is not considered acceptable to eat the exact same breakfast, lunch and dinner for all 28 days. You need a variety of nutrients and the different fruits, veggies, nuts, seeds and animal foods provide different things that are good for your body. Changing things around should be minimal.

• As noted previously, I've chosen to eliminate gluten and non-cultured dairy from this plan. You should not substitute any ingredients in this plan with ingredients that contain gluten or non-cultured dairy.

• The meal schedule assumes that you are starting on a Monday and that you work or are busier on Monday through Friday. For example, the first 5 days of the plan have simple or grab-and-go breakfasts, but the 6th and 7th days usually have slightly more involved breakfast recipes that might be easier to make on a weekend. If this is not the case for you, you can move the days around to fit your schedule better, or substitute as outlined above.

FOOD SOURCING

MEAT SOURCING

When buying meat, local meats that are pasture-raised with sustainable or regenerative methods are preferable to any commercially produced meat source. In fact, even if the farm isn't certified organic, it's probably better than organic meat that is commercially produced and shipped from somewhere else.

However, organic and non-organic meats from the supermarket are acceptable in this program if you cannot find or afford the pasture-raised meats. In general, for beef and poultry, the preference should be like this (from best to worst):

Pasture-raised and local, pasture-raised and non-local, organic non-local, non-organic. For fish, wild-caught is always better than farmed.

Let's go through each type of meat in a bit more detail.

Beef

Cows are "ruminant" animals. This basically means that they are able to digest grass. As humans, we are unable to digest grass. However, we are able to get the plentiful nutrients that the sun imparts to the grasses by way of cattle. Cows eat the grass and turn it into nutrients that we are capable of digesting and then we eat the cows and get the nutrients.

Unfortunately, with corn and other grain subsidies as they are, it's much cheaper to feed cows grains and keep them in confined lots than to let them roam and eat fresh grasses. So, most of the meat you find in a grocery store is from cows that have not been fed their natural diet of grass (at least for the last few months of fattening). This makes the cows sick, alters the fat content of the meat, and results in a whole host of other things that are not good for the animal or for the resulting beef.

The quantities of meat in this plan are not huge and you'll get more taste and more nutrients from grass-fed beef. So, when buying beef, buy as close to the top of the following list as you can afford:

Local, grass-fed, pastured beef: If you can find a local farmer that raises grass-fed cattle, go in with a friend and by a half of a cow and stock your freezer with good meat. You may be able to find one by going to your local farmers market or searching on the internet for farmers in your area. This will be a seasonal thing and may not be a possibility if you are looking to complete this 28-day plan in a specific timeframe.

Grass-fed beef delivery: Programs like ButcherBox will deliver grass-fed beef to your door every month.

I've personally tried this and loved it. It's high-quality meat that is 100% grass-fed. We typically keep a ButcherBox affiliate link because we use it ourselves. Check the resources page

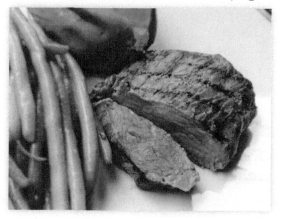

on the website (www.28daystoclean.com/resources) at this page number to see if we still have one.

Grass-fed beef from the grocery store: This is actually just as good as ButcherBox. If you can find 100% grass-fed beef in your local supermarket, that is a good choice. Make sure it says "100% grass-fed" because some have started calling it "grass-fed" even if it is finished in a feed lot with corn for a few months. You'll definitely be able to find good options at stores like Trader Joe's, Sprouts, and Whole Foods, but even larger supermarket chains are starting to carry ground beef and other cuts in a small grass-fed section.

Organic beef: If you can't get grass-fed, the next best would be the standard organic beef. It may be grain-fed or at least grain-finished, but it will be fed with organic feed and won't have all the worst antibiotics. This is still a good option.

Non-organic, standard beef: If you can't afford the options above, you can buy regular beef. It's still going to be better than a calorie-counting, boxed food diet and it still meets the 90/10 requirements.

Chicken, Eggs and Pork

The guidelines are very similar for chicken (and chicken eggs) and pork, but these animals don't eat grass like cows do. You still want to look for local chicken and pork that are "pasture-raised" instead of animals that have been raised in a confined operation.

You'll often see terms like "natural", "free-range", "vegetarian diet" and more when you buy these meats. Unfortunately, these terms aren't very well-regulated. For instance, "free-range" chickens have to have access to the outdoors, but it's often not the same as the picture that the term "free-range" might give you in your head. It can be nothing more than a tiny door to a small yard that is never used by hundreds or even thousands of chickens.

Chickens are often still not allowed to roam and eat the bugs and various other things they would naturally eat from the ground.

Local farmers integrating chickens, cattle, crops, and other animals will have the best chickens and chicken eggs.

When purchasing chicken, eggs, or pork, just like with beef, aim to buy as high on the following list as possible:

Local, pastured-raised: Farmers are allowed to process their own chickens (up to a certain number per year). So, you may find fresh or frozen pastured chickens at farmers markets or farm stores in your area. This is the best-tasting chicken ever.

For eggs, you may even be able to find a hobbyist with a few hens that sells excess eggs. Ask around in your neighborhood and see if someone is selling fresh eggs. The difference in yolk color between a pastured

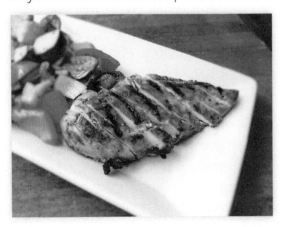

chicken egg and even an organic mass-produced egg is extremely noticeable.

Chicken and pork delivery: Programs like ButcherBox also offer pastured chicken and heritage pastured pork. You can also get chicken from places like Thrive Market. Check the resource page for a link (www.28daystoclean.com/resources) or research other delivery programs.

Organic chicken, eggs, and pork from the supermarket: The next best would be the standard organic chicken, organic chicken eggs, and organic pork you can find in just about any supermarket.

Non-organic, standard chicken: If you can't afford the options above, you can buy regular chicken, eggs, and pork.

Fish

Fish is pretty simple. Wild fish is preferred over farmed fish.

Again, for the most part, it's not a deal-breaker for this plan though. Do your best to avoid farmed fish and stick with wild fish as much as possible. It tastes better and has a better nutritional profile.

Where I live, the Seattle area, wild-caught fish is not difficult to obtain. However, I know it can be much more difficult and expensive to get wild-caught fish such as salmon in areas further from the coast.

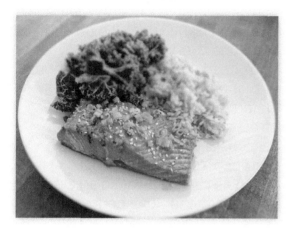

PRODUCE SOURCING

Locally-grown produce is preferable even if it isn't certified organic because produce that has to be picked early in order to be transported is of inferior nutritional quality. Organic (non-local) is next best, and non-organic is last but still acceptable.

If your budget or limited selection does not allow for all organic produce, you should try to buy organic versions of any produce that has difficult to wash surfaces or edible outer surfaces.

Leafy greens, bell peppers, strawberries, apples, pears, and tomatoes are all examples of produce that do not have a removable peel or are typically prepared in a way that removes the outer surface.

Avocados, onions, and pineapple all have outer layers that get removed and are less harmful if purchased as conventional.

COOKING FATS AND OILS

You won't find canola oil, margarine, hydrogenated fats, soybean oil, or corn oil in any of the recipes.

You'll be cooking with butter, extra-virgin olive oil, avocado oil, and coconut oil for the most part. For butter, follow similar guidelines as for sourcing beef (grass-fed). For avocado and olive oil, buy it in a dark or opaque container to avoid light damage.

FOOD SOURCING SUMMARY

In general, you want to go with the most local and unprocessed version of the food you can possibly get. However, the more important point of this process is to switch to eating food rather than food-like substances. So, while grass-fed beef and butter are superior to grain-fed beef and butter, they are both superior to boxed Lean Cuisines with 77 ingredients. Do the best you can with your food sourcing but don't make it a point of failure.

RELAXATION, DIGESTION, AND SLEEP

Most of us live pretty busy and stressful lives, and it's probably unrealistic of me to ask you to change that. Some of you are parents with kids in sports, professionals with demanding jobs, and you have things pulling you in many directions.

I'm not going to try to tell you that you need 9-10 hours of sleep per day, 1 hour of mindful meditation, 1 hour of exercise, and weekly massages in order to be healthy. I mean, if you can do all of that, please do so! But, most of us don't have time for that.

I could go on and on about how our fast-paced lifestyle isn't healthy or I can give you some reasonable and realistic strategies to mitigate this undeniable fact. I'm going to go with the latter.

THE PROBLEM

There are many interconnecting issues with a stressful, busy lifestyle, but these are the main problems, in my opinion:

Stress Response

Our stress hormones still function based on an environment that we no longer inhabit. The stress hormones (such as cortisol and adrenaline) essentially increase blood sugar when you are under stress. Long ago, when stress often involved the need to run for your life, this was perfect. Now, stress can exist with similar hormone responses when you're sitting in your car driving down the highway at 80 mph and someone cuts you off. Clearly, you don't need the blood sugar response at that point, but you get it anyway. Unfortunately, with our lifestyle, stress that can produce hormone responses can be essentially "chronic". Your job or overall schedule can keep you in an elevated cortisol state for long periods of time. This creates a problem of excess blood sugar which leads to fat storage. Elevated stress hormones also work to shut down "unneeded" processes, one of which is digestion. Which brings us to the next item.

Digestion

Your digestive system is designed to work in a relaxed state. When your body is in a stress state, resources are diverted away from digestion to deal with the stress. So, in a stress state, your body's ability to digest food is compromised. Even when we don't have constant and chronic stress and elevated cortisol levels from a difficult job, we often eat on the go and don't take the time to relax around meals. Inhaling a meal while doing 20 other things can seriously compromise your ability to digest that food. Digesting your food is key to overall body function (including thyroid and other systems necessary for weight management). It's impossible for me to overstate the key role that digestion plays in your health.

So, to summarize, stress compromises digestion and increases blood sugar when it really isn't needed. As discussed, the ideal solution for this would be to stop living such a lifestyle. We could

Eat Real Food

The first thing that can help is to eat a nutrient-dense, whole food diet like the one you are about to eat for the next 28 days. You can imagine that dumping refined carbs and sugar on top of already elevated blood sugar is even worse.

Eating a moderate carbohydrate diet with real, whole foods that your digestive system recognizes will go a long way toward mitigating (or at least not propagating) the stress

> "
> ...*stress compromises digestion and increases blood sugar when it really isn't needed.*
> "

all move to France and take long lunches and shorter work weeks. Who's with me?

THE SOLUTIONS

Just in case you decide not to move to France, I've put together a few ideas for minimizing the effects of stress on your overall health and particularly on your ability to digest the healthy food you'll be eating. I mean, how horrible would it be to eat all this healthy food and not get every last benefit of it?

response. You're already good to go with this 4 week plan you're about to start.

Relax Around Meals

I can hear some of you yelling at me through this book: "I barely have time to go to the bathroom at work, much less eat a meal in peace". If that's *truly* the case, you can ignore this one. I simply ask that you give it consideration.

Instead of eating your lunch while answering email, could you take just

15 minutes to eat it on a park bench or somewhere that brings some sense of relaxation? I'm not talking about a 90-minute lunch here. I'm just talking about 15 minutes of peace and quiet to let your body focus on digesting food. This goes for all meals. Any time you can find around meals to breathe and relax is going to be good for your digestion.

Sleep Well

Of course, getting *more* sleep would be great for your health. If you can't do that, at least make sure you get the maximum amount of sleep you can while you're in your bed.

One of the things that is common these days is too much screen time before bed. The blue light from the screens disrupts your melatonin production (a hormone that regulates sleep).

The last thing you want to do is go to bed and lay there for an hour or more without sleeping. Now you're getting nothing done and you're not getting the rest you need. In fact, you might even be stressing about how you're going to be so tired tomorrow.

So, here are a few ways to mitigate this particular issue:

Reduce Screen Time: Of course reducing screen time is a simple (but maybe not easy) way to reduce blue light exposure before bed. Are you screaming at me through the book again?

Use Night Modes: Many phones, tablets and computers have night

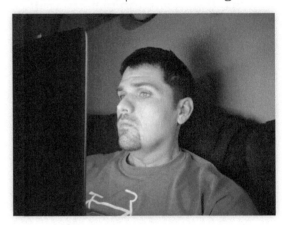

modes that shift the screens to "warmer" light colors so blue light is reduced. This is a great option for reducing blue light exposure from screens.

Blue Light Blocker Glasses: You can buy glasses you can wear at night for blocking blue light. These are usually amber in color and have the advantage of blocking most or all of the sources of blue light (such as regular houselights). See the resources page (www.28daystoclean. com/resources) for some example blue blocker glasses.

Of course, getting in bed at a decent time is a great plan, but don't let screen time ruin it.

WATER AND OTHER BEVERAGES

WATER

You'll be glad to hear that I won't be asking you to calculate your daily water intake based on your body weight. There will be no guzzling down 150 ounces of water to meet the results of some calculation.

You do need to drink water though, and you need to drink plenty of it. What I'd like to do is just tell you "drink plenty of water and let your thirst be your guide".

If that works for you and you aren't tempted to drink 18 sparkling waters per day and hope you are hydrated, then just go with that. I'm serious. No calculation needed. Just drink pure water when you are thirsty.

I know some of you need a goal though, and that's fine. So, here are some basic goals and ways to think about water intake (if you need something other than "drink plenty of water"):

Go by ounces: Shoot for 75 ounces of pure water. You can certainly drink more, but 75 is a decent number to shoot for if you need a goal.

Go by containers: You could also think about 4 containers, 16-20 ounces each. One when you wake up, one mid-morning, one in the afternoon, and one in the evening.

Go by body weight: If you want to do that standard calculation of ½ your body weight in ounces (e.g. 150 lb = 75 ounces), you are welcome to do that as long as it doesn't become a source of stress.

You'll see that the daily schedule reminds you to drink water throughout the day and it is one of your daily action items. Your thirst should help you out here with the action items as the backup.

This is very important for your overall health in so many ways, as you have probably heard many times before.

OTHER BEVERAGES

Pure, plain water should be your primary beverage throughout the day, but not all other beverages are off limits. So, let's go through the major ones so you know what you can do on this plan and what you should avoid.

Alcohol

Alcohol is on the yellow tier in 90/10. So, normally, you can work it into your 10% and have it regularly if you choose to do so. However, for this 28-day plan, you should avoid alcohol so you can really focus on how you feel when eating this way.

So, while alcohol is not normally completely off limits for 90/10, it is for this program.

Coffee and Tea

You may drink coffee and tea on this program. You have to watch what you put in your coffee or tea though.

Black coffee and unsweetened teas are fine in reasonable amounts, which I define as 3 or less cups per day for caffeinated versions. Herbal teas are not usually limited.

Since we are avoiding dairy on this plan, you should not be adding cream to your coffee or tea (although it is normally yellow tier and can be worked in to a 90/10 plan). You also should not be adding anything that is red tier to your drinks (read the ingredients).

You can add unsweetened almond milk, pure stevia or stevia drops, coconut milk, honey, or any other green tier item not mentioned as off limits for this program.

Don't get teas and coffees at coffee shops unless you know the ingredients. The iced teas and lattes and other coffee shop concoctions can be full of sweeteners and dairy and who knows what else. You can most certainly get regular coffee or unsweetened tea though.

It's also important not to use caffeine as a crutch for sagging energy levels for the reasons discussed in the section on relaxation, digestion, and sleep. Caffeine can contribute to that cortisol, chronic stress issue. You may feel like you need it if you are in that cycle right now, but as you eat whole foods, drink water, incorporate some relaxation and sleep, and take care of yourself, you should see that need begin to fade.

Sparkling Water

Someone always asks about sparkling waters such as LaCroix. In my experience, most people who ask if these are ok are drinking many of them as a replacement for regular water. This is not a good idea.

I hesitate to say that sparkling water (unsweetened, just natural flavors) is ok for this program, but as long as you are not replacing regular water intake with it, it is acceptable.

It should be used in small quantities and without affecting your normal hydration.

BEVERAGES SUMMARY

In summary, you should plan to drink plenty of pure water, maybe a small to moderate amount of coffee or tea, and a sparkling water or two if you're so inclined. No alcohol, sugary beverages, sodas, energy drinks, special lattes, or anything else not addressed here.

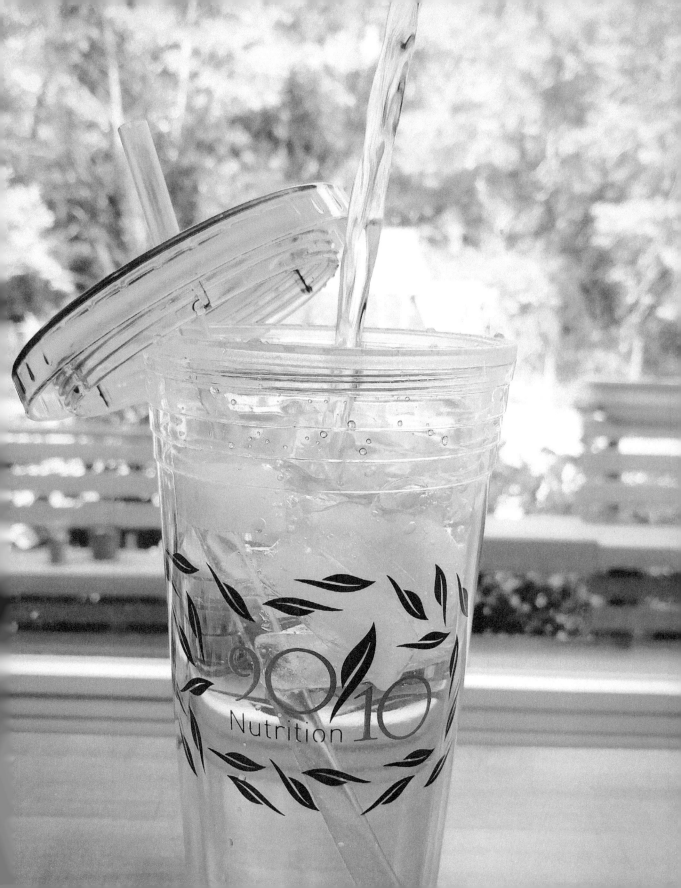

EXERCISE

I highly encourage you to get exercise during your 28 day journey. I'm not going to lay out a specific plan for you to follow in this book because it isn't the focus of the book, but I will give you some thoughts.

Many people get in a mindset where exercise has to be hard or nothing. If you aren't doing burpees at CrossFit then why bother, right? Well, that's just not true. Your body benefits from regular, low aerobic exercise too. Don't get it in the "all or nothing" mindset and compare yourself to the fittest people at the gym. If that IS you, then great. If it's not you, then come up with a different plan.

Here's one of my favorite exercise plans of all time: Grab an audio book that will challenge your brain (learn a new language, study a topic that you don't understand, listen to a perspective you don't agree with) and then simply MOVE for 30-60 minutes per day with that book in your ear. You can run, walk, do stair repeats, do hill repeats, or some combination of all of them. You'll be exercising your body and your mind at the same time.

If you want something a bit more focused on fitness, I think a combination of weight lifting (or bodyweight strength moves) and short intense cardio is one of the most effective combinations ever. You can do something like a 5 or 6 day schedule where you lift for 30 minutes on one body part (chest, back, arms, shoulders, legs) and then finish with 15-20 minutes of interval cardio. Or, you can just incorporate more bodyweight strength moves into your interval cardio routine and make it 30-40 minutes.

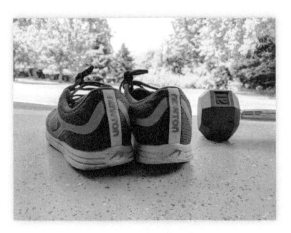

There are just so many options for fitness. You could train for a triathlon or running race, lift, go to CrossFit, walk every day, or take classes at the local gym. Do something that keeps you coming back and doesn't become an unhealthy stress. Just make sure you get some movement!

I'll be reminding you to move throughout the book. Do your best to make it a priority without making it a point of undue stress and worry.

PERSPECTIVE

I could literally write an entire book about how important mindset is when it comes to health. I can't do that here in this section, but just know that I feel it would be impossible for me to overstate the importance of mindset.

If you ignore the advice in this section, my experience tells me that you will have a lower chance of freeing yourself from the diet cycle that so many of us know well.

Here are a few perspectives to help:

Perspective #1

It's about getting rid of "products", not finding better ones. Far too often, I see people focusing on finding healthier products. They think they've

single thing with a label. That would probably be ideal, but I don't think it's necessary. I'm just talking about mindset here. Don't get into a "find a healthier" product mindset. Get into a "eat fewer products and more real foods" mindset.

Perspective #2

Focus on how you feel, not the number on the scale. I know, a few of you just rolled your eyes out loud. I understand your frustration with this perspective, but maybe you should give it a chance this time. Has focusing on the number done you any good?

I think, for most of us, the idea of focusing on how we feel makes

> **" Focus on how you feel, not the number on the scale. "**

found a healthier bag of popcorn or chips, a healthier coffee creamer, a healthier fizzy drink, etc. Get rid of that mindset. Your mindset should be on releasing yourself from the idea that food comes in the form of products. Real food doesn't work like that. Now, that doesn't mean that there aren't "products" out there that are ok and you need to shun every

sense, but it's the execution of it that is difficult. It's much harder to measure how you feel than it is to get on the scale and get the hard data. It requires awareness. You have to actively ponder how you feel throughout the day and take note of your current state. This takes work, but it's worth it.

Awareness is one of the keys to many

aspects of life. Awareness can be the difference between saying something to a loved one that you'll regret later and taking a second to calm down before responding. In the same way, it can make the difference between eating a cookie you aren't even hungry for just because it was offered and saying "no thanks".

Here's an idea: Set an hourly or bi-hourly reminder in your phone that just says, "how do you feel right now?" Use this reminder to take inventory. This will help you fill out your daily worksheet. In most cases, the weight loss results will follow as well.

Perspective #3

You're not restricted, you're free. Sure, we've "restricted" wheat and most dairy on this plan as well as all processed food and refined sugar.

Unfortunately, this feels like half of the grocery store is off limits and that feels restrictive.

This is a newly created problem though. Most of the things restricted on this plan were not even available 100 years ago, and most of us haven't even tried but a fraction of the real foods available on this planet.

Almost every real food (fruits, nuts, vegetables, meats, seeds, and more) is available to you. You're not held hostage by the food companies and their diet food labels in order to be healthy. You are free to roam the world of real food and enjoy.

You're not restricted by calorie counting, macronutrient counting, or even super strict portion sizes. You can just eat real food.

COMMON QUESTIONS

Inevitably, you're going to run into some obstacles during your 28 days on this program.

Maybe you'll end up staying late at work and you won't be able to cook the meal that is on the plan. Maybe your kids will have to go to a birthday party and you'll give in to the cake tempation. Maybe you'll be feeling hungry all the time. Maybe you'll be the opposite and you'll feel like you can't eat all of the food.

If any of these are the case, just use the guidance below.

Q: What do I do if I mess up and eat something that isn't on the plan?

This is an important question and will come up for many of you. Over the course of a 28 day plan, it's very possible that you'll get a bit off plan here or there. It's IMPERATIVE that you take this piece of advice seriously: Just get right back on the plan. There's literally nothing good that comes from beating yourself up about it. There's nothing good that comes from starving for 3 days to try to make up for it. There's nothing to do but get right back on plan. That's all. Trust me.

Q: What do I do if I'm still hungry all the time?

Excellent question. This is NOT a starvation plan. If you are truly hungry, eat a bit more. It's almost impossible to determine portions for a book like this and make sure that they will satisfy everyone's needs. With that said, the key here is if you are truly hungry. Did you drink enough water today? Are you just bored? Is it habit or actual hunger? Try to listen to your body and see if you can tell. Be honest with yourself, and if you're truly still hungry, eat more!

Q: What do I do if I can't eat all the food?

Another excellent question. The answer to this one is similar to the last question. If you truly are full and don't want more food, you don't have to eat more food. This is NOT a starvation plan though. Eating less to lose weight is not the answer. You don't have to be hungry all the time for this to work, so don't fall into that crash diet mindset trap.

DAILY ACTION ITEMS CHECKLIST

- ☐ Drink water throughout the day

- ☐ MOVE! Get 30 minutes or more of intentional movement

- ☐ Check tomorrow's schedule to make sure you are ready

- ☐ Fill out your daily worksheet

- ☐ Check in with the online group or a friend who is doing this with you

- ☐ Limit blue light exposure in the evening and get to bed on time

- ☐ Eat meals in a relaxed environment to aid digestion

- ☐ Do your best

- ☐ Give yourself some grace if you mess up

- ☐ Believe in yourself at least just a little

- ☐ Practice awareness (are you actually hungry, do you feel good or bad, do you actually want it, are you thirsty)

> ⓘ **NOTE:** You can get a printable checklist and worksheet online at www.28daystoclean.com/resources

DAILY WORKSHEET

Hydration

I drank plenty of water today: ☐ Yes ☐ No

NOTES: _____

Exercise

I moved my body today: ☐ Yes ☐ No

NOTES: _____

Eating

I followed the plan today: ☐ Yes ☐ No ☐ Mostly

I ate at the following times: _____ _____ _____ _____ _____

Hunger level between meals (1-10 with 10 being the most hungry): _____

Satisfaction level with meals (1-10 with 10 being very satisfied): _____

NOTES: _____

Energy Levels

Energy level and various times of the day (1-10 with 10 being highest energy):

___ ___ ___ ___ ___ ___ ___ ___ ___ ___ (example: 10:30am, 7)

Summary

I give myself a score of _____ for today (1-10 with 10 being the best)

My overall energy level today was a ____ (1-10 with 10 being the best)

The hardest part for me today was: _____

My biggest wins today were: _____

Tomorrow, I could do the following things better: _____

_____

_____

General Notes: _____

_____

_____

_____

_____

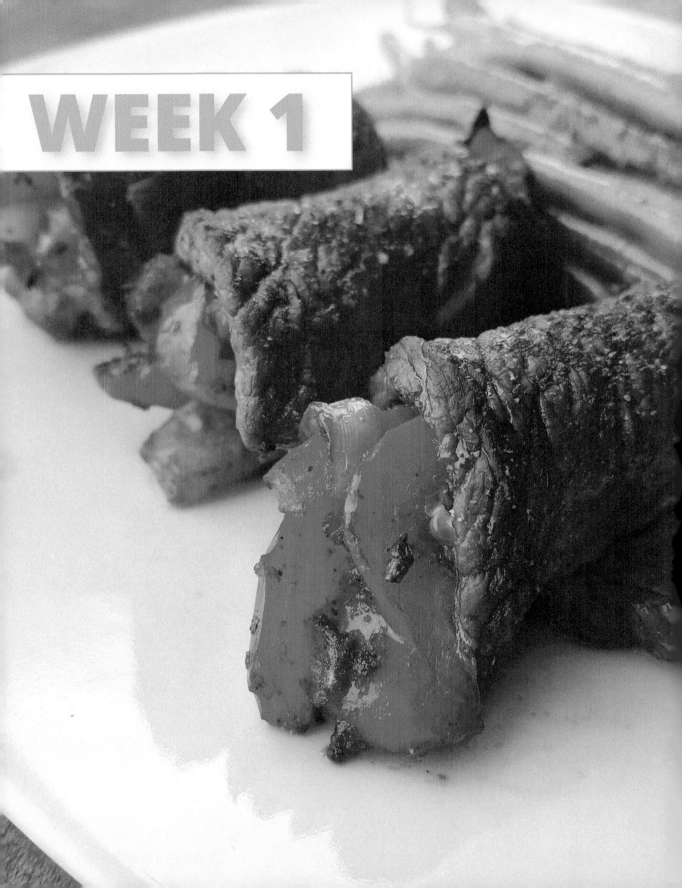

WEEK 1 SCHEDULE

	Upon Waking	Breakfast	Midmorning	Lunch	Afternoon	Dinner
Day 1	12-16 oz water	Overnight Oats (pg. 99)	Snack + water (optional)	Salad (pg. 113) + 2 hard-boiled eggs (pg. 179)	Snack (pg. 181) + water	Steak, Brussels Sprouts, Rice (pg. 117)
Day 2	12-16 oz water	Scramble or Omelet (pg. 100)	Snack + water (optional)	Salad (pg. 113) + leftover steak	Snack (pg. 181) + water	Chicken and Brown Rice (pg. 118)
Day 3	12-16 oz water	Overnight Oats (pg. 99)	Snack + water (optional)	Leftover Chicken and Brown Rice	Snack (pg. 181) + water	One Pan Salmon and Broccoli (pg. 121)
Day 4	12-16 oz water	Coconut Berry Smoothie (pg. 103)	Snack + water (optional)	Leftover Chicken and Brown Rice	Snack (pg. 181) + water	Fajita Rollups and Green Beans (pg. 122)
Day 5	12-16 oz water	Overnight Oats (pg. 99)	Snack + water (optional)	Salad (pg. 113) + leftover Fajita Rollups	Snack (pg. 181) + water	One Pan Chicken and Carrot Fries (pg. 125)
Day 6	12-16 oz water	Scramble or Omelet (pg. 100)	Snack + water (optional)	Leftover Chicken and Carrot Fries	Snack (pg. 181) + water	Taco Rice Bowls (pg. 126)
Day 7	12-16 oz water	Coconut Berry Smoothie (pg. 103)	Snack + water (optional)	Leftover Taco Rice Bowls	Snack (pg. 181) + water	Pork Chops, Sweet Potatoes, Asparagus (pg. 129)

The day or night before your first day, do the following to make sure you're ready for the week. Some of the stuff is optional and could be made on the day you need it rather than before the week starts. However, anything you do from this section will set you up for success during the week. The more prepared you are, the less likely you are to order take out.

Make Hard-Boiled Eggs

You're going to need hard-boiled eggs for some salads as well as snack options. Use the recipe on page 179. If you don't plan to use them for snacks, you only need to make 2 eggs. If you plan to use them for snacks, make 2 in addition to the amount you need for snacks this week.

Make Dressing Packs

You'll need dressing for 3 salads this week. You can pick one or multiple dressings from the dressings section of this book (starting on page 172) or you can use Primal Kitchen dressings (you can get them at thrivemarket. com/9010nutrition). You may also use any other dressing that is completely green tier with no gluten or dairy.

If you are making a dressing from the recipes in this book, I suggest packaging it in single serving containers or an easy pourable container. Make it as easy to grab as possible. If you are taking your lunches to work, for example, single-serve containers may work best.

Make Salads and Chop Veggies

You'll have 3 salads this week for lunch and the rest will mostly be intentional leftovers from your dinners. I suggest you chop the veggies for your salads and package them in 1 gallon resealable bags or other resealable containers. This is especially important if you work outside the home. You need to set yourself up for success by having everything ready to go. Prepping a salad in the morning before work is possible but it's very easy for this to end up being a point of failure. You can remove that possibility by having everything ready. Use the recipe on page 113 to make up your salads.

You'll also want to chop your veggies for your scrambles/omelets. You can make the entire scramble to heat up in the mornings or just chop the veggies and store in the fridge. Either way is fine. I prefer to just chop the veggies and then cook the scramble or omelet fresh in the morning. It really doesn't take much time if the veggies are ready to go. Use the recipe on page 100 and the calendar for week 1 to see what quantities you need.

Make Overnight Oats

Overnight fridge oatmeal is on the breakfast list for 3 days this week. So, make them up before the week starts and they'll make an easy to grab breakfast during the first week. See page 99 for the recipe.

Make Brown Rice

You'll need approximately 2 cups of cooked brown rice (1 cup dry) for this week. You can make brown rice in a rice cooker, on the stove top, or in the Instant Pot. Use the recipe on page 178.

Save the rice in one container or 4 individual containers for the week.

NOTE: You also need 1 cup of uncooked brown rice for the Chicken and Brown Rice recipe on day 2, but you will not cook this ahead of time.

Snacks

Check out the snack options on page 181 and do any prep you need to. If you're going to be taking them to work, packaging them into single-serve bags/containers that you grab in the morning is a really good plan.

Other Notes

If you're super busy and have very little time to cook, you might want to look ahead at the meals for this week and do any other little things you can. None of the meals are particularly difficult or time-consuming, but mixing up spices and pre-chopping veggies can save time if you need it.

🛈 REMINDER

You can find helpful additional resources such as printables and links online at www.28daystoclean.com/resources (or simply use the QR code to the right).

MEAT

- ☐ Sirloin Steak (grass-fed) - 8 oz
- ☐ Chicken Breast (pasture-raised) - 16 oz
- ☐ Salmon Fillet (wild) - 6 oz
- ☐ Skirt or Flank Steak (grass-fed) - 1 lb
- ☐ Ground Beef (grass-fed) - 1 lb
- ☐ Pork Chop (pasture-raised) - 4-6 oz

CANNED

- ☐ Chicken Broth - 1 cup
- ☐ Coconut Milk - 1 cup
- ☐ Black Beans - 1 can, 15 oz

OTHER

- ☐ Honey
- ☐ Bottled Minced Garlic
- ☐ Salsa (optional, for taco rice bowls and eggs)
- ☐ Hot Sauce (optional, for eggs)
- ☐ Almond Butter - 2 Tbsp

ADDITIONAL ITEMS

- ☐ Ingredients for chosen snacks
- ☐ Ingredients for chosen salad dressings
- ☐ _____
- ☐ _____
- ☐ _____
- ☐ _____
- ☐ _____
- ☐ _____
- ☐ _____
- ☐ _____

PRODUCE

- ☐ Mixed Salad Greens - 9 cups total
- ☐ Avocado, Haas - 4 total
- ☐ Brussels Sprouts - 1 cup
- ☐ Onion - 2
- ☐ Spinach - 1 cup
- ☐ Red Bell Pepper - 3
- ☐ Cucumber - 1
- ☐ Tomatoes - 3
- ☐ Carrots - 2 lbs
- ☐ Mushrooms, sliced - 1 pint (allows extra for salads)
- ☐ Parsley, fresh - small bunch (optional)
- ☐ Green Onions - 2
- ☐ Broccoli Florets - 2 cups
- ☐ Green Beans - 1/2 lb
- ☐ Kale - 3 cups
- ☐ Lemons - 2 (for lemon juice)
- ☐ Cilantro - 1 bunch
- ☐ Sweet Potato - 1 small
- ☐ Asparagus - 1 bunch

FROZEN

- ☐ Frozen Berries (or fresh) - 4 cups
- ☐ Frozen Peas - 1/2 cup
- ☐ Frozen corn - 1 cup
- ☐ _____
- ☐ _____
- ☐ _____
- ☐ _____
- ☐ _____
- ☐ _____
- ☐ _____

DRY GOODS

- ☐ Brown Rice, 2 cups (dry amount)
- ☐ Rolled Oats (gluten free) - 2 cups
- ☐ Flax Meal or Chia Seeds - 3 Tbsp
- ☐ Sesame Seeds - 2 tsp

DAIRY & EGGS

- ☐ Eggs - 8 + any for snacks
- ☐ Greek or Regular Yogurt (full fat, plain) - 1 cup
- ☐ Almond Milk, unsweetened - 3 1/4 cups
- ☐ Butter (grass-fed if possible)

SPICES AND STAPLES

- ☐ Extra Virgin Olive Oil
- ☐ Balsamic Vinegar
- ☐ Salt
- ☐ Pepper
- ☐ Italian Seasoning
- ☐ Sesame Oil
- ☐ Bragg Liquid Aminos
- ☐ Coconut Oil
- ☐ Chili Powder
- ☐ Cumin
- ☐ Onion Powder
- ☐ Garlic Powder
- ☐ Oregano
- ☐ Paprika
- ☐ Curry Powder
- ☐ _____
- ☐ _____
- ☐ _____
- ☐ _____
- ☐ _____

Welcome to day 1! If you did your prep, you should be all set for breakfast, lunch, and snacks. If you didn't do your prep, don't panic. You can switch some things around and still make it work.

SCHEDULE

Upon Waking: 12-16 oz pure water

Breakfast: Overnight Oats. You should have this all prepped and ready to grab from the fridge. This breakfast is full of healthy fats and proteins from the yogurt, almond milk and flax. It has whole grain carbs and fiber from the oats, and antioxidants from the berries.

Midmorning: Drink water throughout the morning. Snack is optional depending on your schedule and if you are truly hungry.

Lunch: Mixed Green Salad (see page 113) with 2 Hard-boiled Eggs and choice of dressing. I almost didn't put a salad on the first day because of the stigma surrounding salads and dieting. But, it's not going to be all salads on this plan and you can definitely handle a salad on day 1 (uh, and maybe on day 2 as well). Once we start cooking some awesome dinners, you'll be having tasty leftovers.

Afternoon: Drink water throughout the afternoon. Pick one snack from the options on page 181.

Dinner: Balsamic Steak, Brussels Sprouts, and Brown Rice (see page 117). Speaking of awesome dinners, the steak is incredible tonight. Make sure you let it marinate for at least 20 minutes.

NOTE: You'll save half the steak for tomorrow's lunch.

← **NOTE:** You can get a printable shopping list online at www.28daystoclean.com/resources

Welcome to day 2. I want you to remember to be aware today. Be aware of yourself and your thoughts, feelings, and decisions.

Sometimes, poor nutrition decisions are made simply because we aren't aware of our choices. We grab something out of habit. We do something because others are doing it. We assume we want it because it's unhealthy.

The candy jar in the break room, the donuts someone brought in, or the vending machine can all be nearly mindless decisions. But, if you take a moment to step back and evaluate the situation for a minute, you may find that you aren't even hungry, you don't even really want that thing, or you don't care because you're more concerned with doing something good for yourself. Take a moment to be aware.

SCHEDULE

Upon Waking: 12-16 oz pure water

Breakfast: 3 egg Veggie Scramble (or omelet) with Avocado (see page 100). This is one of my favorite power breakfasts. I usually make it as a scramble because it's a bit easier, but either way is fine. Don't skip the veggies.

Midmorning: Drink water throughout the morning. Snack is optional depending on your schedule and if you are truly hungry.

Lunch: Mixed Green Salad (see page 113) with steak and choice of dressing. You're going to use some of that awesome steak from last night to make your salad amazing.

Afternoon: Drink water throughout the afternoon. Pick one snack from the options on page 181.

Dinner: Chicken and Brown Rice (see page 118). I love this one because I make it all at once in the Instant Pot. If you don't have one, you can still do it, but it really is a breeze in the "IP".

NOTE: The recipe makes 3 servings so you'll have two lunches ready to go for following days.

Are you remembering your water intake? As discussed, it doesn't need to be 2 gallons of water, but you need to be consistent and hydrate. It makes such a difference in how you feel and move, so don't skimp on the water.

SCHEDULE

Upon Waking: 12-16 oz pure water

Breakfast: Overnight Oats. Breakfast is super easy again this morning. Just grab and go from the fridge.

Midmorning: Drink water throughout the morning. Snack is optional depending on your schedule and if you are truly hungry.

Lunch: Leftover Chicken and Brown Rice. I hope you enjoyed last night's dinner recipe because that's what is on the menu for lunch today. It heats up well. You can always do another salad if you like, but having a warm lunch to change things up is a plus in my book.

Afternoon: Drink water throughout the afternoon. Pick one snack from the options on page 181.

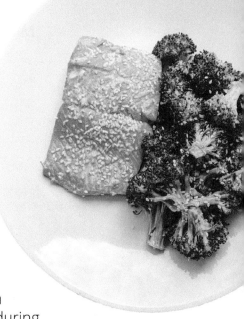

Dinner: One Pan Salmon and Sesame Broccoli (see page 121). Dinner all goes on one pan in the oven. Easy. "Sheet Pan Meals", as they are often called, make great dinners with very little clean up. If you use parchment paper on the sheet pan, it's even easier. We'll use these sheet pan meals several times during this program.

Have you been getting some movement in this week? A walk every day? Remember, it doesn't have to be a 2 hour run or an intense lifting session. It most certainly can be intense workouts if you like, but those aren't required. Just having a goal of getting 30 minutes of focused movement is going to make you feel amazing.

SCHEDULE

Upon Waking: 12-16 oz pure water

Breakfast: Coconut Berry Smoothie (see page 103). Your breakfast this morning has nuts, coconut milk, berries, and more. Use a little honey if you want it a bit sweeter, but I recommend you try it without honey to see.

Midmorning: Drink water throughout the morning. Snack is optional depending on your schedule and if you are truly hungry.

Lunch: Leftover Chicken and Brown Rice.

Afternoon: Drink water throughout the afternoon. Pick one snack from the options on page 181.

Dinner: Steak Fajita Rollups and 7-minute Green Beans (see page 122).

NOTE: You'll be making 2 servings of the steak fajita rollups tonight so you have one serving for a salad topping tomorrow.

One thing you may notice as we go through this program is that you won't typically find carbohydrate-heavy meals for both lunch and dinner. For instance, on day 2, we had chicken and brown rice for dinner. That dish is fairly heavy with rice, but lunch that day was a salad with protein. Then, on days 3 and 4 where the lunch was leftover chicken and brown rice, the dinners were lower in carbs. This is strategic. This isn't a low carb or a "keto" plan, but it's far too easy to end up with bread, pasta, rice, and oatmeal all in one day. Our goal here is to be balanced but not to an exact number. It's just about eating whole foods and not sticking more to one type than to other types. We want a healthy variety of everything from the green tier (greens, whole grains, healthy fats, quality protein). This is nothing like counting macros. It's just eating real food with variety and balance.

SCHEDULE

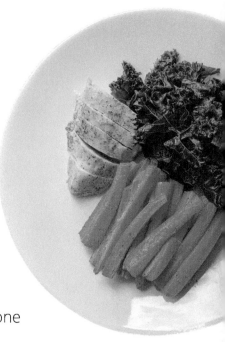

Upon Waking: 12-16 oz pure water

Breakfast: Overnight Oats. Use up your last serving of overnight oats today.

Midmorning: Drink water throughout the morning. Snack is optional depending on your schedule and if you are truly hungry.

Lunch: Mixed Green Salad (see page 113) with leftover steak fajita rollups and choice of dressing. Just top your salad with your leftover fajita rollups from last night.

Afternoon: Drink water throughout the afternoon. Pick one snack from the options on page 181.

Dinner: One Pan Chicken with Carrot Fries and Steamed Kale (see page 125). The carrot fries are so good and the steamed kale is my wife's absolute favorite. She has to have it at least once per week.

NOTE: The recipe makes 2 servings (except the kale) so you'll have lunch for tomorrow.

You're almost through with week 1. I wish I could ask you how you feel and hear your response myself, but take a minute and ask yourself right now - How *do* I feel? Think about it all day today. Are you wishing you weren't on a diet? Are you hungry all day? Be honest with yourself and let yourself feel however you feel about it. I urge you to take the time to be aware of your body and how you are feeling instead of relying on the scale to tell you if you are succeeding.

SCHEDULE

Upon Waking: 12-16 oz pure water

Breakfast: 3 egg Veggie Scramble (or omelet) with Avocado (see page 100). Feel free to change things up a bit. Hot sauce, salsa, different veggies, etc.

Midmorning: Drink water throughout the morning. Snack is optional depending on your schedule and if you are truly hungry.

Lunch: Leftover Chicken and Carrot Fries. You can add a salad if you want and use the chicken more as a topping (as well as the carrots), if you prefer.

Afternoon: Drink water throughout the afternoon. Pick one snack from the options on page 181.

Dinner: Taco Rice Bowls (see page 126). I don't know about you, but I love Mexican food. If I'm going to eat out at a "fast food" type of place, Chipotle is my choice. So, I love these taco rice bowls from tonight's dinner menu. Enjoy.

NOTE: The recipe makes 3 servings so you'll have two lunches ready to go for following days.

You've made it to the last day of week 1. Congratulations. Take some time today to reflect back on what went well this week and what didn't go so well. Celebrate the things that went well. Evaluate the things that didn't go so well. Why didn't they go well? Can you do something to set yourself up better for success this week?

Speaking of setting yourself up for success, don't forget to take a look at week 2 prep today so you are ready to go for next week.

SCHEDULE

Upon Waking: 12-16 oz pure water

Breakfast: Coconut Berry Smoothie (see page 103).

Midmorning: Drink water throughout the morning. Snack is optional depending on your schedule and if you are truly hungry.

Lunch: Leftover Taco Rice Bowl.

Afternoon: Drink water throughout the afternoon. Pick one snack from the options on page 181.

Dinner: Curry Grilled Pork Chops with Baked Sweet Potatoes and Asparagus (see page 129).

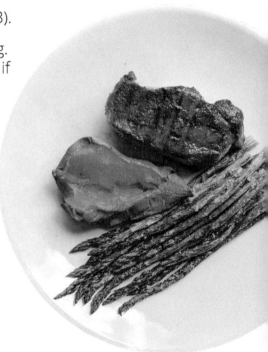

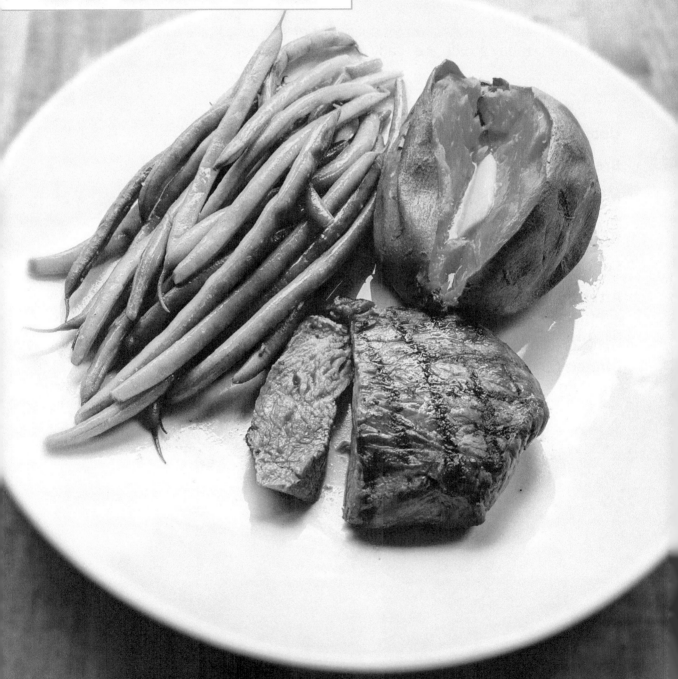

WEEK 2 SCHEDULE

	Upon Waking	Breakfast	Midmorning	Lunch	Afternoon	Dinner
Day 8	12-16 oz water	Overnight Oats (pg. 99)	Snack + water (optional)	Leftover Taco Rice Bowl	Snack (pg. 181) + water	Ryan's Beef Chili (pg. 130)
Day 9	12-16 oz water	Breakfast Berry Crisp (pg. 102)	Snack + water (optional)	Leftover Beef Chili	Snack (pg. 181) + water	Steak, Sweet Potatoes, Green Beans (pg. 133)
Day 10	12-16 oz water	Overnight Oats (pg. 99)	Snack + water (optional)	Salad (pg. 113) + leftover steak	Snack (pg. 181) + water	Sweet Potato Shepherd's Pie (pg. 134)
Day 11	12-16 oz water	Breakfast Berry Crisp (pg. 102)	Snack + water (optional)	Leftover Shepherd's Pie	Snack (pg. 181) + water	Mahi-Mahi, Brown Rice, Broccoli (pg. 137)
Day 12	12-16 oz water	Overnight Oats (pg. 99)	Snack + water (optional)	Salad (pg. 113) + leftover mahi-mahi	Snack (pg. 181) + water	Steak Stir Fry with Brown Rice (pg. 138)
Day 13	12-16 oz water	Scramble or Omelet (pg. 100)	Snack + water (optional)	Leftover Steak Stir Fry, Brown Rice	Snack (pg. 181) + water	Garlic Ranch Chicken and Veggies (pg. 141)
Day 14	12-16 oz water	Breakfast Berry Crisp (pg. 102)	Snack + water (optional)	Leftover Ranch Chicken and Veggies	Snack (pg. 181) + water	Teriyaki Salmon, Brown Rice, Steamed Kale (pg. 142)

The day or night before your first day of week 2, do the following to make sure you're ready for the week. Some of the stuff is optional and could be made on the day you need it rather than before the week starts.

Make Hard-Boiled Eggs

You only need hard-boiled eggs this week if you choose to use them as snacks. If you choose to use other snack options, you can skip this. If you choose to use eggs as a snack, use the recipe on page 179 and make as many as you need.

Make Dressing Packs

You'll need dressing for 2 salads this week. You can pick one or multiple dressings from the dressings section of this book (starting on page 172) or you can use Primal Kitchen dressings (you can get them at thrivemarket. com/9010nutrition). You may also use any other dressing that is completely green tier with no gluten or dairy.

If you are making a dressing from the recipes in this book, I suggest packaging it in single serving containers as suggested in week 1.

Make Salads and Chop Veggies

You'll have 2 salads this week for lunch and the rest will mostly be intentional leftovers from your dinners. I suggest you chop the veggies for your salads and package them in 1 gallon resealable bags or other resealable containers as suggested in week 1.

You'll also want to chop your veggies for your scrambles/omelets. You can make the entire scramble to heat up in the mornings or just chop the veggies and store in the fridge. Either way is fine. I prefer to just chop the veggies and then cook the scramble or omelet fresh in the morning. It really doesn't take much time if the veggies are ready to go. Use the recipe on page 100 and the calendar for week 2 to see what quantities you need.

Make Overnight Oats

Overnight fridge oatmeal is on the breakfast list for 3 days this week. So, make them up before the week starts and they'll make an easy to grab breakfast during the week. See page 99 for the recipe.

Make Breakfast Berry Crisp

You also have a berry crisp for breakfast 3 days this week. This is something I would make up before as well. You can either make it all in one pan and then just reheat servings on a plate, or you can make it in individual ramekins and either bake and then reheat or even bake each morning fresh. Use the recipe on page 102.

Make Brown Rice

You'll need approximately 2 cups of cooked brown rice (1 cup dry) for this week. You can make brown rice in a rice cooker, on the stove top, or in the Instant Pot. Use the recipe on page 178.

Save the rice in one container or 4 individual containers for the week.

Snacks

Check out the snack options on page 181 and do any prep you need to. If you're going to be taking them to work, packaging them into single-serve bags/containers that you grab in the morning is a really good plan.

Other Notes

If you're super busy and have very little time to cook, you might want to look ahead at the meals for this week and do any other little things you can. None of the meals are particularly difficult or time-consuming, but mixing up spices and pre-chopping veggies can save time if you need it.

ⓘ REMINDER

You can find helpful additional resources such as printables and links online at www.28daystoclean.com/resources (or simply use the QR code to the right).

MEAT

- [ ] Sirloin Steak (grass-fed) - 8 oz
- [ ] Chicken Breast (pasture-raised) - 2 (4-6 oz each)
- [ ] Mahi-Mahi Fillets - 2 (4-6 oz each)
- [ ] Skirt or Flank Steak (grass-fed) - 1/2 lb
- [ ] Ground Beef (grass-fed) - 1 lb
- [ ] Salmon Fillet - 1 (6 oz)

CANNED

- [ ] Vegetable Broth - 3/4 cup
- [ ] Tomato Paste - 1 Tbsp
- [ ] Diced Tomatoes - 2 cans (15 oz each)
- [ ] Red Kidney Beans - 1 can (15 oz)

OTHER

- [ ] Honey
- [ ] Bottled Minced Garlic
- [ ] Pure Maple Syrup
- [ ] Pickled Jalapenos - about 10 slices needed

ADDITIONAL ITEMS

- [ ] Ingredients for chosen snacks
- [ ] Ingredients for chosen salad dressings
- [ ] _____
- [ ] _____
- [ ] _____
- [ ] _____
- [ ] _____
- [ ] _____
- [ ] _____

PRODUCE

- [ ] Mixed Salad Greens - 6 cups total
- [ ] Avocado, Haas - 2
- [ ] Celery - 1 stalk (use extra for snacks)
- [ ] Onion - 2
- [ ] Basil, fresh - small bunch
- [ ] Bell Pepper - 3
- [ ] Cucumber - 1
- [ ] Tomatoes - 2
- [ ] Carrots - 2 medium (use extras for snacks)
- [ ] Mushrooms, sliced - 1 pint
- [ ] Parsley, fresh - small bunch
- [ ] Sugar Snap Pea Pods - 1/2 lb
- [ ] Broccoli Florets - 1 1/2 cups
- [ ] Green Beans - 1/2 lb
- [ ] Kale - 2 cups
- [ ] Zucchini - 1
- [ ] Green Onions - 1-2
- [ ] Sweet Potato - 2
- [ ] Ginger, fresh - small piece
- [ ] Spinach - 1/2 cup
- [ ] Purple or Sweet Potatoes - 8 oz
- [ ] Baby Carrots - 8 oz
- [ ] Lemon - 1 (for lemon juice)

FROZEN

- [ ] Frozen Berries (or fresh) - 5 cups
- [ ] Frozen Peas - 1/2 cup
- [ ] _____
- [ ] _____
- [ ] _____
- [ ] _____

DRY GOODS

- [ ] Brown Rice, 1 cup (dry amount)
- [ ] Rolled Oats (gluten free) - 2 cups
- [ ] Flax Meal Or Chia Seeds - 3 Tbsp
- [ ] Sesame Seeds - 1/2 Tbsp
- [ ] Walnuts - 1/2 cup
- [ ] Pecans - 1/2 cup
- [ ] Cornstarch - 1 tsp

DAIRY & EGGS

- [ ] Eggs - 3 + any for snacks
- [ ] Greek or Regular Yogurt (full fat, plain) - 1 cup
- [ ] Almond Milk, unsweetened - 1 1/4 cups
- [ ] Butter (grass-fed if possible)

SPICES AND STAPLES

- [ ] Extra Virgin Olive Oil
- [ ] Salt
- [ ] Pepper
- [ ] Sesame Oil
- [ ] Bragg Liquid Aminos
- [ ] Coconut Oil
- [ ] Chili Powder
- [ ] Onion Powder
- [ ] Paprika
- [ ] Cinnamon
- [ ] Cardamom or Nutmeg
- [ ] Vanilla Extract - 1 Tsp
- [ ] Rosemary
- [ ] Thyme
- [ ] Dried Chives
- [ ] Parsley
- [ ] Dill

Welcome to day 8! You've made it to week 2. Hopefully you've been utilizing your daily action items checklist and worksheets so you can keep track of how you feel. If you haven't, get a piece of paper right now and just do a little inventory before you embark on your second week.

SCHEDULE

Upon Waking: 12-16 oz pure water

Breakfast: Overnight Oats. Your breakfast for today should be familiar. Routine is good. We'll change it up a bit this week, but we'll also keep some things the same. We'll try to find that perfect balance of new and familiar.

Midmorning: Drink water throughout the morning. Snack is optional depending on your schedule and if you are truly hungry.

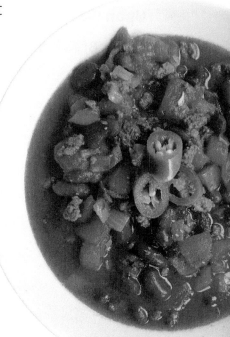

Lunch: Leftover Taco Rice Bowl. Speaking of familiar, you should have another taco rice bowl leftover from last week. If you're anything like me, you're looking forward to that.

Afternoon: Drink water throughout the afternoon. Pick one snack from the options on page 181.

Dinner: Ryan's Beef Chili (see page 130). For dinner, you'll treat yourself to the best chili in the world. I mean, I suppose that is not a settled matter in everyone's mind, but I think you'll like it.

NOTE: You'll be making 2 servings with this recipe. One will be for your lunch tomorrow. The recipe calls for ½ lb of ground beef. You need ½ lb of ground beef for day 10 as well. So, brown the whole pound today to make day 10 easier.

← **NOTE:** You can get a printable shopping list online at www.28daystoclean.com/resources

REMINDER: MOVE! Just a little movement every day will do wonders. You don't need a Fitbit or a CrossFit membership (those are fine, too). Just be kind to your body and move it around. It was meant to move. As I have mentioned, it's also a great time to exercise your mind. I know you probably exercise your mind in many ways throughout the day, but this movement time can be a time where you can learn something that excites you. Kill 2 birds with one stone (or two stones with one bird, if you're Chuck Norris) and better your body and mind.

SCHEDULE

Upon Waking: 12-16 oz pure water

Breakfast: Breakfast Berry Crisp. You should have this ready from prep, but if not, see page 102.

Midmorning: Drink water throughout the morning. Snack is optional depending on your schedule and if you are truly hungry.

Lunch: Leftover Chili. If you're heating this up at work, guard it so none of your coworkers steal it.

Afternoon: Drink water throughout the afternoon. Pick one snack from the options on page 181.

Dinner: Sirloin Steak, Baked Sweet Potatoes, 7-minute Green Beans (see page 133). Dinner is a simple 1-2-3 Eat! recipe with steak, sweet potatoes, and 7-minute green beans. I think we already learned about 7-minute green beans in week 1, so I won't reiterate how IMPORTANT the 7-minutes is...too much.

NOTE: You'll save half of the steak to go with your lunch tomorrow as well.

For most people, the hardest thing on the daily action items list is probably relaxing around meals to aid digestion. I know it is. In fact, I might have just had to take a break before writing this because I was trying to eat my lunch while working. I know the struggle with it firsthand. We live in a world that promotes the idea that you have to be busy all the time to be worthy. I'm actively trying to remember that my worth isn't based on how busy I am. I hope you will too. This is your extra reminder to take some time today to eat in peace if you can.

SCHEDULE

Upon Waking: 12-16 oz pure water

Breakfast: Overnight Oats. Use your second serving of overnight oats this morning. Just grab and go from the fridge.

Midmorning: Drink water throughout the morning. Snack is optional depending on your schedule and if you are truly hungry.

Lunch: Mixed Green Salad (see page 113) with leftover steak and choice of dressing. Just pile your leftover steak on the salad for some healthy protein. You can warm it up or leave it cold.

Afternoon: Drink water throughout the afternoon. Pick one snack from the options on page 181.

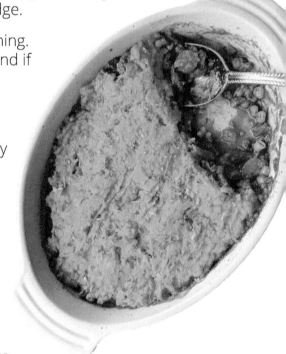

Dinner: Sweet Potato Shepherd's Pie (see page 134). Dinner is comfort food! This doesn't take too long to make and it comes out so good and so hearty.

NOTE: The recipe makes 2 servings, so you'll have lunch for tomorrow.

I just imagine my body being so happy when I put food like this into it. I imagine it taking everything in and saying, "I know what to do with that, I'll put that over here, that will help with that, we've been low on that." When I put processed junk food in, I imagine it having to work so hard to separate out the good stuff and make use of it. You're helping your body so much by giving it stuff it recognizes and knows how to utilize!

SCHEDULE

Upon Waking: 12-16 oz pure water

Breakfast: Breakfast Berry Crisp. Bring on the antioxidants and healthy fats. You should have this ready, but if not, see page 102.

Midmorning: Drink water throughout the morning. Snack is optional depending on your schedule and if you are truly hungry.

Lunch: Leftover Shepherd's Pie. Your leftovers should make for a fantastic lunch today.

Afternoon: Drink water throughout the afternoon. Pick one snack from the options on page 181.

Dinner: Basil Butter Mahi-Mahi, Brown Rice, and Broccoli (see page 137). Mahi-mahi is one of my favorite types of fish. It's also known as "dolphin" (not the porpoise) or "dorado". This was always on the menu growing up in Florida. If you can't find mahi-mahi, you can substitute other white fish. Remember your sourcing hierarchy (wild caught is always preferred).

NOTE: You're making 2 servings of the mahi-mahi so you can have it with another amazing salad tomorrow.

Reset your mind. You're not depriving yourself of foods, you're freeing yourself from the prison of fake food. You're freeing yourself from the constant cycle of being hungry, being low on energy, and always needing to "diet". I'm not saying it is easy to break yourself free. I'm not saying it's just a simple switch. It takes time and practice, but it's worth the time and practice to reset your mind. Be aware of your self talk and thoughts about food, and remind yourself of your freedom when you find the same old thoughts repeating. You are worth your effort and patience.

SCHEDULE

Upon Waking: 12-16 oz pure water

Breakfast: Overnight Oats. Use your final serving of the overnight oats this morning.

Midmorning: Drink water throughout the morning. Snack is optional depending on your schedule and if you are truly hungry.

Lunch: Mixed Green Salad (see page 113) with leftover mahi-mahi and choice of dressing. The mahi-mahi goes well on a nice salad. Enjoy.

Afternoon: Drink water throughout the afternoon. Pick one snack from the options on page 181.

Dinner: Steak Stir Fry with Brown Rice (see page 138).

NOTE: The recipe makes 2 servings, so you'll have lunch for tomorrow.

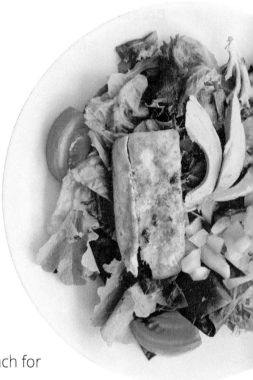

You're almost to the halfway point of this program. Give yourself some credit for making it this far even if you haven't been perfect. Celebrate today or tomorrow with some relaxation time, a movie, spa time, shopping or whatever else you like to reward yourself with other than food that is going to make you feel "blech". Find a different way to celebrate, but definitely celebrate a bit.

SCHEDULE

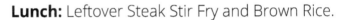

Upon Waking: 12-16 oz pure water

Breakfast: 3 egg Veggie Scramble (or omelet) with Avocado (see page 100).

Midmorning: Drink water throughout the morning. Snack is optional depending on your schedule and if you are truly hungry.

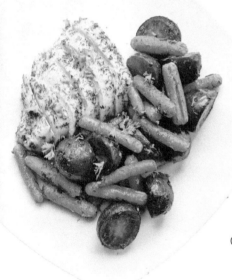

Lunch: Leftover Steak Stir Fry and Brown Rice.

Afternoon: Drink water throughout the afternoon. Pick one snack from the options on page 181.

Dinner: One Pan Garlic Ranch Chicken and Veggies (see page 141). This is another one pan meal but with a ranch flavor this time. It gets rave reviews in the 90/10 world, so I think you'll enjoy it.

NOTE: The recipe makes 2 servings, so you'll have one for lunch tomorrow.

This is the last day of week 2! If you haven't been keeping up with your daily worksheets and action items, take some time to think back on the week. What did you do well? What could you do better?

Also, don't forget to take a look at week 3 prep today so you are ready to go for next week.

SCHEDULE

Upon Waking: 12-16 oz pure water

Breakfast: Breakfast Berry Crisp. Use your final serving of this tasty crisp this morning. You probably have this ready from your weekly prep, but if not, see page 102.

Midmorning: Drink water throughout the morning. Snack is optional depending on your schedule and if you are truly hungry.

Lunch: Leftover Ranch Chicken and Veggies.

Afternoon: Drink water throughout the afternoon. Pick one snack from the options on page 181.

Dinner: Teriyaki Salmon with Brown Rice and Steamed Kale (see page 142). This is different than your typical lemon or broiled salmon and should be a welcome change.

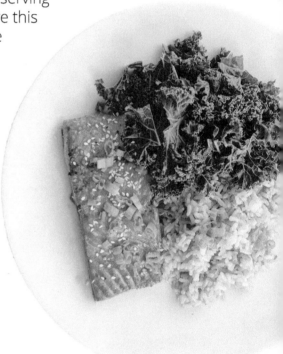

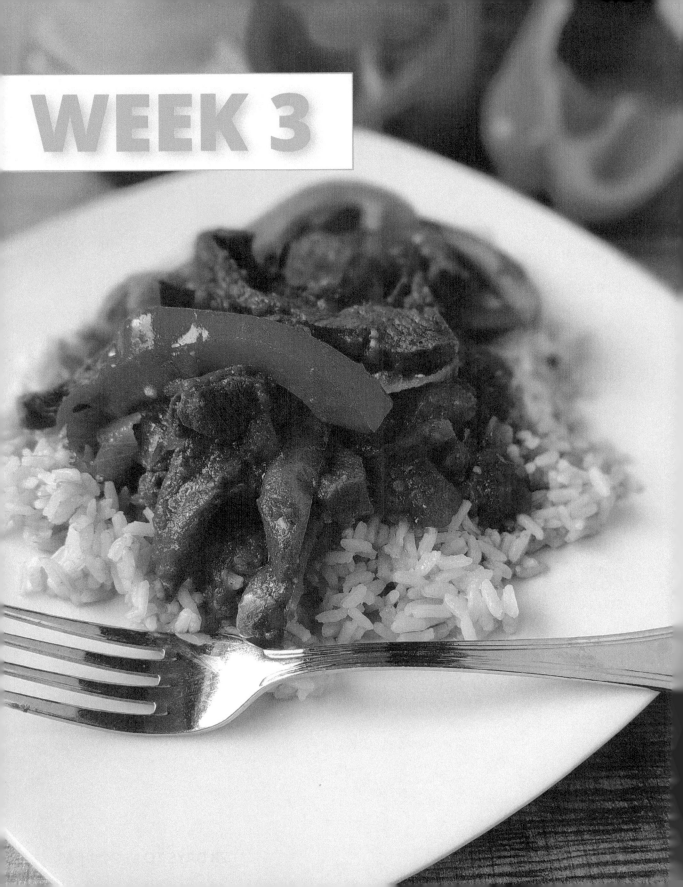

WEEK 3 SCHEDULE

	Upon Waking	Breakfast	Midmorning	Lunch	Afternoon	Dinner
Day 15	12-16 oz water	Bacon and Egg Muffins (pg. 106)	Snack + water (optional)	Salad (pg. 113) + 2 hard-boiled eggs (pg. 179)	Snack (pg. 181) + water	Beef and Pepper Soup (pg. 145)
Day 16	12-16 oz water	Almond Milk Hot Oatmeal (pg. 105)	Snack + water (optional)	Leftover Beef and Pepper Soup	Snack (pg. 181) + water	Balsamic Chicken and Veggies (pg. 146)
Day 17	12-16 oz water	Bacon and Egg Muffins (pg. 106)	Snack + water (optional)	Leftover Balsamic Chicken and Veggies	Snack (pg. 181) + water	Mexican Lasagna (pg. 149)
Day 18	12-16 oz water	Almond Milk Hot Oatmeal (pg. 105)	Snack + water (optional)	Leftover Mexican Lasagna	Snack (pg. 181) + water	Orange Salmon, Brown Rice, Green Beans (pg. 150)
Day 19	12-16 oz water	Bacon and Egg Muffins (pg. 106)	Snack + water (optional)	Leftover Mexican Lasagna	Snack (pg. 181) + water	Burgers with Baked Chili Fries (pg. 153)
Day 20	12-16 oz water	Coconut Flour Pancakes (pg. 109)	Snack + water (optional)	Orange Salmon Lettuce Wraps	Snack (pg. 181) + water	One Pan Sausage and Apples (pg. 154)
Day 21	12-16 oz water	Almond Milk Hot Oatmeal (pg. 105)	Snack + water (optional)	Leftover One Pan Sausage and Apples	Snack (pg. 181) + water	Slow Cooker Pepper Steak (pg. 157)

The day or night before your first day of week 3, do the following to make sure you're ready for the week. Some of the stuff is optional and could be made on the day you need it rather than before the week starts.

Make Hard-Boiled Eggs

You're going to need hard-boiled eggs for some salads as well as snack options. Use the recipe on page 179. If you don't plan to use them for snacks, you only need to make 2 eggs. If you plan to use them for snacks, make 2 in addition to the amount you need for snacks this week.

Make Dressing Packs

You'll need dressing for just 1 salad this week. You can pick a dressing from the dressings section of this book (starting on page 172) or you can use Primal Kitchen dressings (you can get them at thrivemarket. com/9010nutrition). You may also use any other dressing that is completely green tier with no gluten or dairy.

If you are making a dressing from the recipes in this book, I suggest packaging it in single serving containers as suggested in previous weeks.

Make Salads and Chop Veggies

You'll have 1 salad this week for lunch and the rest will mostly be intentional leftovers from your dinners. I suggest you chop the veggies for your salads and package them in 1 gallon resealable bags or other resealable containers. This is especially important if you work outside the home. You need to set yourself up for success by having everything ready to go. Prepping a salad in the morning before work is possible but it's very easy for this to end up being a point of failure. You can remove that possibility by having everything ready. Use the recipe on page 113 to make up your salads.

Make Almond Milk Hot Oatmeal Packs

This week, you'll be having almond milk hot oatmeal for breakfast 3 times. You are welcome to use the overnight fridge oats from weeks 1 and 2 if you prefer, but this will give you a little change. You'll want to go ahead and mix up the dry parts of this recipe during prep so all you have to do is heat it with the almond milk in the morning. See the recipe on page 105.

Make Bacon and Egg Muffins

You have egg muffins for breakfast 3 times this week. These are pretty easy to make in muffin tins and then reheat on the morning you are scheduled to have them. You'll have 3 egg muffins per meal, so the recipe is intended to make 9 total. Find the recipe on page 106.

Make Brown Rice

You'll need approximately 1 1/2 cups of cooked brown rice (3/4 cup dry) for this week. You can make brown rice in a rice cooker, on the stove top, or in the Instant Pot. Use the recipe on page 178.

You don't need any rice until about day 18 though (day 4 of this week). So, you don't have to do this before the week starts. I just suggest you make it all at once, either before the week or on day 18.

Snacks

Check out the snack options on page 181 and do any prep you need to. If you're going to be taking them to work, packaging them into single-serve bags/containers that you grab in the morning is a really good plan.

Other Notes

If you're super busy and have very little time to cook, you might want to look ahead at the meals for this week and do any other little things you can. None of the meals are particularly difficult or time-consuming, but mixing up spices and pre-chopping veggies can save time if you need it.

> **ⓘ REMINDER**
>
> You can find helpful additional resources such as printables and links online at www.28daystoclean.com/resources (or simply use the QR code to the right).

MEAT

- ☐ Sirloin Steak (grass-fed) - 10 oz
- ☐ Chicken Breast (pasture-raised) - about 1 lb total
- ☐ Uncured Bacon (no sugar in ingredients) - 6 oz
- ☐ Uncured Chicken Sausage (no sugar) - 2 links
- ☐ Ground Beef (grass-fed) - 1 lb
- ☐ Salmon Fillets - 2 (4-6 oz each)

CANNED

- ☐ Beef Broth - 2 cups
- ☐ Crushed or Petite Diced Tomatoes - 2 cans (15 oz)
- ☐ Diced Tomatoes - 1 can (15 oz)
- ☐ Black Beans - 1 can (15 oz)
- ☐ Black Olives, sliced - 2 oz (optional)

OTHER

- ☐ Honey
- ☐ Bottled Minced Garlic
- ☐ Pure Maple Syrup
- ☐ Almond Butter - 2 Tbsp
- ☐ Corn Tortillas - 8
- ☐ Salsa - 1 cup (no sugar in ingredients)
- ☐ Apple Sauce, unsweetened - 1/4 cup

ADDITIONAL ITEMS

- ☐ Ingredients for chosen snacks
- ☐ Ingredients for chosen salad dressings
- ☐ _____

PRODUCE

- ☐ Mixed Salad Greens - 3 cups total
- ☐ Avocado, Haas - 1
- ☐ Riced cauliflower - 1 cup
- ☐ Onion - 2
- ☐ Red Onion - 2
- ☐ Bell Pepper - 5 (mix of colors)
- ☐ Cucumber - 1
- ☐ Tomatoes - 2
- ☐ Carrots, baby - 1/2 lb
- ☐ Mushrooms, Baby Bella - 1 pint
- ☐ Apple (granny smith) - 1
- ☐ Broccoli Florets - 2 cups
- ☐ Green Beans - 1/2 lb
- ☐ Yellow Squash - 1
- ☐ Zucchini - 1
- ☐ Green Onions - 1 (optional)
- ☐ Jalapeno, fresh - 1 (optional)
- ☐ Orange - 1
- ☐ Fresh Berries (for pancakes)
- ☐ Purple or Sweet Potato - 1 small to medium
- ☐ Purple or Sweet Potato - 3/4 lb
- ☐ Leafy Green Lettuce (for burger)
- ☐ Fresh sage (dried is ok)

FROZEN

- ☐ Frozen Berries (or fresh) - 3 cups
- ☐ Frozen Diced Onions - 1/2 cup (or 1/2 of a fresh one)
- ☐ Frozen Diced Carrots - 1/2 cup (or fresh carrots diced)
- ☐ Frozen Bell Pepper Mix - 1 cup (or 1 fresh pepper)
- ☐ Frozen Corn - 1 cup

DRY GOODS

- ☐ Brown Rice, 3/4 cup (dry amount)
- ☐ Rolled Oats (gluten free) - 2 cups
- ☐ Flax Meal Or Chia Seeds - 3 Tbsp
- ☐ Walnuts - 1/4 cup
- ☐ Coconut Flour - 1/2 cup
- ☐ Baking Soda - 1/2 tsp

DAIRY & EGGS

- ☐ Eggs - 12 + any for snacks
- ☐ Almond Milk, unsweetened - 2 1/2 cups
- ☐ Butter (grass-fed if possible)

SPICES AND STAPLES

- ☐ Extra Virgin Olive Oil
- ☐ Salt
- ☐ Pepper
- ☐ Bragg Liquid Aminos
- ☐ Coconut Oil
- ☐ Chili Powder
- ☐ Onion Powder
- ☐ Oregano
- ☐ Cinnamon
- ☐ Dried Basil
- ☐ Paprika
- ☐ Garlic Powder
- ☐ Cumin
- ☐ Cayenne Pepper
- ☐ Ground Coriander
- ☐ Balsamic Vinegar
- ☐ _____
- ☐ _____
- ☐ _____

Welcome to day 15! Week 3 of 4 is upon us. Whether you've rocked every day so far or made a million "mistakes", you are here reading day 15 and continuing on. This is most definitely a process that takes time and everything you do moves you forward. Just being here ready to take on week 3 is moving you forward.

SCHEDULE

Upon Waking: 12-16 oz pure water

Breakfast: 3 Bacon and Egg Muffins. You should have this ready to reheat from prep. If not, find the recipe on page 106.

Midmorning: Drink water throughout the morning. Snack is optional depending on your schedule and if you are truly hungry.

Lunch: Mixed Green Salad (see page 113) with 2 Hard-boiled Eggs and choice of dressing. Since you don't have leftovers from yesterday, we're going to do a tasty and familiar salad for lunch today. It's the only one of the week, but it will be refreshing and good. You should have some hard-boiled eggs to go on the salad from your preps for the week.

Afternoon: Drink water throughout the afternoon. Pick one snack from the options on page 181.

Dinner: Beef and Pepper Soup with a side of Broccoli (see page 145). I love the flavor of this soup and it's hearty despite the fact that it's pretty low in carbohydrates.

NOTE: This recipe makes at least 2 servings, so you'll have one leftover for lunch tomorrow. Also, take note of the ground beef instructions in the recipe.

← **NOTE:** You can get a printable shopping list online at www.28daystoclean.com/resources

This is your weekly reminder to move. Remember that getting a bit of movement in every day (intense, light, medium or whatever works for you) is so essential. Get outside and into the fresh air if you can, but get some exercise either way!

SCHEDULE

Upon Waking: 12-16 oz pure water

Breakfast: Almond Milk Hot Oatmeal. You should have this mostly ready from prep, but see page 105 for what to do this morning to finish preparing this. This is your first day of hot oatmeal unless you opted to stick with the overnight fridge oats. This can be a nice change from the cold oats.

Midmorning: Drink water throughout the morning. Snack is optional depending on your schedule and if you are truly hungry.

Lunch: Leftover Beef and Pepper Soup. As always, you can do a salad if you don't have any leftover, but the recipe makes a bit more than 2 servings, so you probably have plenty.

Afternoon: Drink water throughout the afternoon. Pick one snack from the options on page 181.

Dinner: Balsamic Grilled Chicken and Veggies (see page 146). This is like a sheet pan meal for the grill because everything gets the same marinade and pretty much cooks all together. In fact, you could do this as a sheet pan meal if you don't want to use the grill.

NOTE: There is a 1 hour marinate time on this dinner recipe. You'll also save half of this for lunch tomorrow.

Are you getting to bed on time? You know, I really need emojis and gifs right now. I need to be on a message with you and wagging my finger with the perfect gif. Ha! But seriously, are you doing your best to get some relaxation time, proper sleep, and recovery? I hope so!

SCHEDULE

Upon Waking: 12-16 oz pure water

Breakfast: 3 Bacon and Egg Muffins. You should have this ready to reheat from prep. If not, find the recipe on page 106.

Midmorning: Drink water throughout the morning. Snack is optional depending on your schedule and if you are truly hungry.

Lunch: Leftover Balsamic Chicken and Veggies.

Afternoon: Drink water throughout the afternoon. Pick one snack from the options on page 181.

Dinner: Mexican Lasagna (see page 149). I may have mentioned that I love Mexican food. This lasagna is no exception. It's easy and it's fun and unique.

NOTE: The recipe makes 3 servings, so you'll have lunch for two days from the leftovers.

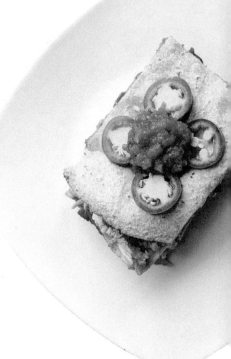

Your body is thanking you for the last 2-1/2 weeks. I know it is. Think of all the things you'll be able to do when your body works well. Think of all the things you can do when you feel GOOD! Keep going.

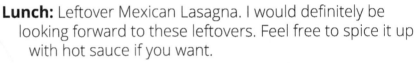

SCHEDULE

Upon Waking: 12-16 oz pure water

Breakfast: Almond Milk Hot Oatmeal. You should have this mostly ready from prep, but see page 105 for what to do this morning to finish preparing this.

Midmorning: Drink water throughout the morning. Snack is optional depending on your schedule and if you are truly hungry.

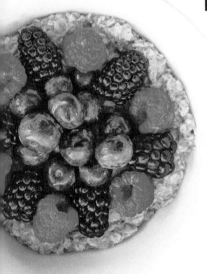

Lunch: Leftover Mexican Lasagna. I would definitely be looking forward to these leftovers. Feel free to spice it up with hot sauce if you want.

Afternoon: Drink water throughout the afternoon. Pick one snack from the options on page 181.

Dinner: Orange Salmon, Brown Rice, 7-minute Green Beans (see page 150). Another tasty, simple "1-2-3 Eat! Meal".

NOTE: You're making 2 servings of the salmon (not the sides) for use in lettuce wraps in a lunch.

Everyone has different struggles and different backgrounds. I'm sure some of you doing this program came in with tons of knowledge and just needed a little help. Others of you may have come straight from eating fast food and packaged foods every day. Some of you are comfortable in the kitchen and some of you struggle. Some of you love food and others struggle to eat enough.

What I want you to know is that you don't need to be ashamed of where you came from or where you are currently. You are here making changes whether they are small for you or big for you. You're moving forward. Be proud of that as we finish up week 3.

SCHEDULE

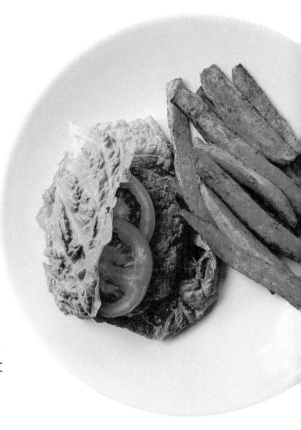

Upon Waking: 12-16 oz pure water

Breakfast: 3 Bacon and Egg Muffins. You should be using up your last 3 muffins today for breakfast.

Midmorning: Drink water throughout the morning. Snack is optional depending on your schedule and if you are truly hungry.

Lunch: Leftover Mexican Lasagna.

Afternoon: Drink water throughout the afternoon. Pick one snack from the options on page 181.

Dinner: Lettuce Wrapped Burgers with Baked Chili Fries (see page 153). These are messy but oh so tasty.

The scale is a thief of joy. I don't know how many times I've spent a few weeks putting good food into my body, exercising, getting rest, drinking my water, and felt absolutely amazing, only to find that scale hadn't moved. Ugh! I hate that. It can absolutely be deflating if you don't have your mind right. The scale is ONE piece of data. Don't let it negate all the other data. If you feel good, have more energy, and your clothes fit better, the scale is not telling the whole story. Don't let it dominate the story with its one data point.

SCHEDULE

Upon Waking: 12-16 oz pure water

Breakfast: Coconut Flour Pancakes with Berries and Maple Syrup (see page 109). These are a bit trickier to flip than regular pancakes, but they have such good flavor. Give them a try!

Midmorning: Drink water throughout the morning. Snack is optional depending on your schedule and if you are truly hungry.

Lunch: Salmon Lettuce Wraps (no recipe page). Just use your leftover orange salmon from day 18. Fill some lettuce leaves with salmon and any veggie toppings you wish. Try onion, tomato, avocado, and any other chopped veggies that you think would taste good.

Afternoon: Drink water throughout the afternoon. Pick one snack from the options on page 181.

Dinner: One Pan Sausage and Apples (see page 154). Another sheet pan meal with a bit of a twist.

NOTE: The recipe makes 2 servings, so you'll have lunch for tomorrow.

This is the last day of week 3! It's inventory time. If you've been keeping your daily worksheets, take a minute to go back through them and review. If you haven't, just take some time to reflect and think about how the week went and how you can make adjustments (if needed) for this week.

SCHEDULE

Upon Waking: 12-16 oz pure water

Breakfast: Almond Milk Hot Oatmeal. Use up your last serving of oatmeal for breakfast today. See page 105 for instructions if you need a reminder.

Midmorning: Drink water throughout the morning. Snack is optional depending on your schedule and if you are truly hungry.

Lunch: Leftover One Pan Sausage and Apples.

Afternoon: Drink water throughout the afternoon. Pick one snack from the options on page 181.

Dinner: Slow Cooker Pepper Steak with Brown Rice (see page 157). I love the slow cooker as much or more than I love sheet pan dinners!

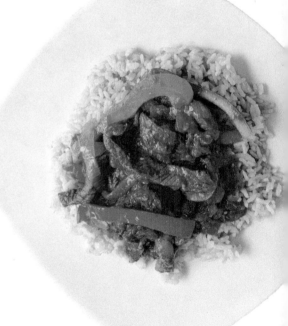

NOTE: The recipe makes 2 servings, so you'll have lunch for tomorrow.

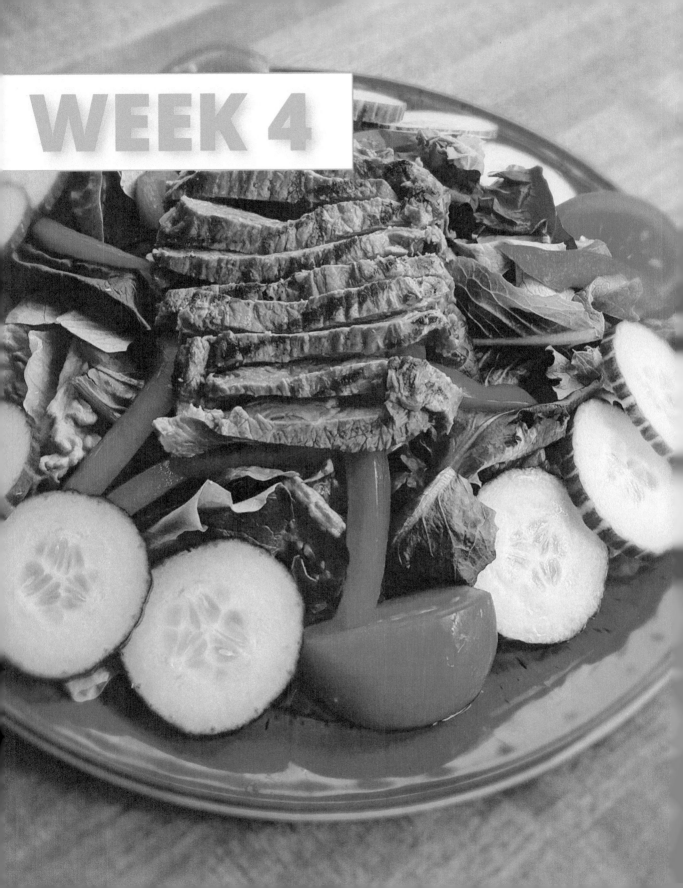

WEEK 4

WEEK 4 SCHEDULE

	Upon Waking	Breakfast	Midmorning	Lunch	Afternoon	Dinner
Day 22	12-16 oz water	Almond Milk Hot Oatmeal (pg. 105)	Snack + water (optional)	Leftover Pepper Steak	Snack (pg. 181) + water	Pork Fried Rice (pg. 158)
Day 23	12-16 oz water	Scramble or Omelet (pg. 100)	Snack + water (optional)	Leftover Pork Fried Rice	Snack (pg. 181) + water	Butter Pan Steak, Kale, Quinoa (pg. 161)
Day 24	12-16 oz water	Almond Milk Hot Oatmeal (pg. 105)	Snack + water (optional)	Salad (pg. 113) + leftover steak	Snack (pg. 181) + water	White Chicken Chili (pg. 162)
Day 25	12-16 oz water	Coconut Berry Smoothie (pg. 103)	Snack + water (optional)	Leftover Pork Fried Rice	Snack (pg. 181) + water	One Pan Salmon and Broccoli (pg. 121)
Day 26	12-16 oz water	Almond Milk Hot Oatmeal (pg. 105)	Snack + water (optional)	Leftover White Chicken Chili	Snack (pg. 181) + water	Lettuce-Wrapped Carnitas Tacos (pg. 165)
Day 27	12-16 oz water	Coconut Flour Pancakes (pg. 109)	Snack + water (optional)	Salad (pg. 113) + leftover carnitas	Snack (pg. 181) + water	Thai Chicken Soup (pg. 166)
Day 28	12-16 oz water	Coconut Berry Smoothie (pg. 103)	Snack + water (optional)	Leftover Thai Chicken Soup	Snack (pg. 181) + water	One Pan Pork and Veggies (pg. 169)

The day or night before your first day of week 4, do the following to make sure you're ready for the week. Some of the stuff is optional and could be made on the day you need it rather than before the week starts.

Make Hard-Boiled Eggs

You only need hard-boiled eggs this week if you choose to use them as snacks. If you choose to use other snack options, you can skip this. If you choose to use eggs as a snack, use the recipe on page 179 and make as many as you need.

Make Dressing Packs

You'll need dressing for 2 salads this week. You can pick one or multiple dressings from the dressings section of this book (starting on page 172) or you can use Primal Kitchen dressings (you can get them at thrivemarket. com/9010nutrition). You may also use any other dressing that is completely green tier with no gluten or dairy.

If you are making a dressing from the recipes in this book, I suggest packaging it in single serving containers as suggested in previous weeks.

Make Your Salads and Chop Your Veggies

You'll have 2 salads this week for lunch and the rest will mostly be intentional leftovers from your dinners. I suggest you chop the veggies for your salads and package them in 1 gallon resealable bags or other resealable containers as suggested in previous

You'll also want to chop your veggies for your scramble/omelet on day 2 of this week (day 23). You can make the entire scramble to heat up in the morning or just chop the veggies and store in the fridge. Either way is fine. I prefer to just chop the veggies and then cook the scramble or omelet fresh in the morning. It really doesn't take much time if the veggies are ready to go. Use the recipe on page 100 to see what quantities you need.

Make Almond Milk Hot Oatmeal Packs

Just like last week, you'll be having almond milk hot oatmeal for breakfast 3 times this week. You'll want to go ahead and mix up the dry parts of this recipe during prep. See the recipe on page 105.

Make Brown Rice

You only need to make brown rice if you don't have an Instant Pot for the Pork Fried Rice on day 2 of this week (Day 23). If you have an Instant Pot, the rice cooks along with the meat in the Instant Pot. If you don't, you will need to cook the rice separately. See the recipe on page 158 and then decide if you want to go ahead and cook rice before the week starts. If you do, use the recipe for brown rice on page 178.

Snacks

Check out the snack options on page 181 and do any prep you need to. If you're going to be taking them to work, packaging them into single-serve bags/containers that you grab in the morning is a really good plan.

Other Notes

If you're super busy and have very little time to cook, you might want to look ahead at the meals for this week and do any other little things you can. None of the meals are particularly difficult or time-consuming, but mixing up spices and pre-chopping veggies can save time if you need it.

ⓘ REMINDER

You can find helpful additional resources such as printables and links online at www.28daystoclean.com/resources (or simply use the QR code to the right).

MEAT

- [ ] Sirloin Steak (grass-fed) - 8 oz
- [ ] Chicken Breasts (pasture-raised) - 1 1/2 lb
- [ ] Pork Chops, boneless (pasture-raised) - 8 oz
- [ ] 1 1/2 lb Pork Tenderloin (pasture-raised)
- [ ] Salmon Fillet - 1 (6 oz)

CANNED

- [ ] Chicken Broth - 4 cups
- [ ] Green Chiles, 1 can, 4 oz
- [ ] Coconut Milk, canned, full fat - 2 cans
- [ ] White Beans (such as cannelini) - 1 can, 15 oz

OTHER

- [ ] Honey
- [ ] Bottled Minced Garlic
- [ ] Pure Maple Syrup
- [ ] Red Curry Paste - 2 tsp
- [ ] Almond Butter - 4 Tbsp
- [ ] Apple Sauce, unsweetened - 1/4 cup

ADDITIONAL ITEMS

- [ ] Ingredients for chosen snacks
- [ ] Ingredients for chosen salad dressings
- [ ] _____
- [ ] _____
- [ ] _____
- [ ] _____
- [ ] _____

PRODUCE

- [ ] Mixed Salad Greens - 6 cups total
- [ ] Avocado, Haas - 2
- [ ] Large Lettuce Leaves - 3 or 4
- [ ] Onion - 3
- [ ] Green Bell Pepper - 1
- [ ] Bell Pepper (any color, for salads and scrambles) - 2
- [ ] Cucumber - 1
- [ ] Tomatoes - 1
- [ ] Carrots - 2 large
- [ ] Mushrooms, sliced - 1 pint
- [ ] Cilantro, fresh - small bunch
- [ ] Berries, fresh (for pancake topping. Or use frozen)
- [ ] Broccoli Florets - 2 cups
- [ ] Snow Peas - 3 oz
- [ ] Kale - 3 cups
- [ ] Bean Sprouts - 1 cup
- [ ] Green Onions - 3-4
- [ ] Sweet Potato - 3/4 lb
- [ ] Ginger, fresh - small piece
- [ ] Spinach - 1/2 cup
- [ ] Brussels Sprouts - 4 oz
- [ ] Baby Carrots - 4 oz
- [ ] Lemon - 1 (for lemon juice)

FROZEN

- [ ] Frozen Berries (or fresh) - 3 cups
- [ ] Frozen Peas - 1/2 cup
- [ ] _____
- [ ] _____
- [ ] _____
- [ ] _____

DRY GOODS

- [ ] Brown Rice, 1 cup (dry amount)
- [ ] Rolled Oats (gluten free) - 2 cups
- [ ] Flax Meal or Chia Seeds - 3 Tbsp
- [ ] Sesame Seeds - 1/2 Tbsp
- [ ] Walnuts - 1/4 cup
- [ ] Coconut Flour - 1/4 cup
- [ ] Quinoa, 1/4 cup (dry amount)
- [ ] Baking Soda, 1/4 tsp

DAIRY & EGGS

- [ ] Eggs - 6 + any for snacks
- [ ] Almond Milk, unsweetened - 4 1/2 cups
- [ ] Butter (grass-fed if possible)

SPICES AND STAPLES

- [ ] Extra Virgin Olive Oil
- [ ] Salt
- [ ] Pepper
- [ ] Sesame Oil
- [ ] Bragg Liquid Aminos
- [ ] Coconut Oil
- [ ] Chili Powder
- [ ] Chipotle chile powder
- [ ] Paprika
- [ ] Cinnamon
- [ ] Thyme
- [ ] Cayenne Pepper
- [ ] Oregano
- [ ] Cumin
- [ ] _____
- [ ] _____
- [ ] _____

Ah...the final week. As you start week 4, I want you to begin thinking about what you'll do after this.

You may have already read the transition section at the back of this section of the book. If you haven't, the beginning of this week is a great time to do that.

The last thing you should do is treat this like a short program that you are just about done with. Now is your chance to make this last! So, read that transition section and take it seriously.

SCHEDULE

Upon Waking: 12-16 oz pure water

Breakfast: Almond Milk Hot Oatmeal. We're sticking with the hot oatmeal this week and you're probably a pro at this one now. The instructions are always on page 105 if you need them.

Midmorning: Drink water throughout the morning. Snack is optional depending on your schedule and if you are truly hungry.

Lunch: Leftover Pepper Steak with Brown Rice. You should have this all set from last night's dinner.

Afternoon: Drink water throughout the afternoon. Pick one snack from the options on page 181.

Dinner: Pork Fried Rice (see page 158). This recipe is very similar in concept to the Chicken and Brown Rice recipe from week 1.

NOTE: You're making 3 servings of this tonight which will set you up nicely for some great lunches over the next couple of days.

⬅ **NOTE:** You can get a printable shopping list online at www.28daystoclean.com/resources

It's time to remind you to get some movement in this week. If you've been getting some exercise every day (or most days) during this program, it probably won't take much convincing. You will have discovered the energy and other benefits that come with regular movement and you'll have no problem doing it just about every day. If that's not you yet, I promise you it's like that if you'll give it a chance. Start small but consistent.

SCHEDULE

Upon Waking: 12-16 oz pure water

Breakfast: 3 egg Veggie Scramble (or omelet) with Avocado (see page 100). Start the day with an easy favorite.

Midmorning: Drink water throughout the morning. Snack is optional depending on your schedule and if you are truly hungry.

Lunch: Leftover Pork Fried Rice. This is one of two servings of leftovers you should have from last night.

Afternoon: Drink water throughout the afternoon. Pick one snack from the options on page 181.

Dinner: Butter Pan Steak with Steamed Kale and Quinoa (see page 161). This method of cooking steak is so amazing. I'll admit, I was a "grill only" kind of guy when it comes to steak until I tried this method. Now, I can hardly decide which I like better.

NOTE: You'll save half of your steak to use as a topping on tomorrow's lunch salad.

Can you see yourself making this type of eating your new normal? Real food and a little planning can do wonders. If you're feeling deprived at this point, it could be that you've slipped into the "diet" mindset and you're not eating enough. If that is the case, eat a bit more and see if you are still feeling deprived. If you're feeling good, just keep right on going.

SCHEDULE

Upon Waking: 12-16 oz pure water

Breakfast: Almond Milk Hot Oatmeal. See page 105 for instructions if you need them.

Midmorning: Drink water throughout the morning. Snack is optional depending on your schedule and if you are truly hungry.

Lunch: Mixed Green Salad (see page 113) with steak and choice of dressing. Just top your salad with your leftover steak from last night.

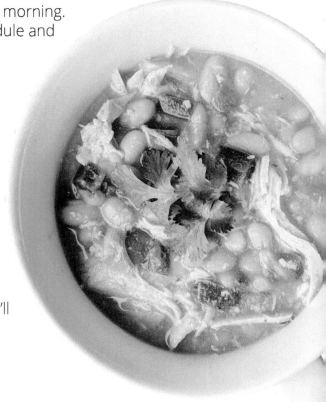

Afternoon: Drink water throughout the afternoon. Pick one snack from the options on page 181.

Dinner: White Chicken Chili (see page 162). You can make this one in the slow cooker or on the stove.

NOTE: The recipe makes 2 servings, so you'll have one lunch from the leftovers.

I want to take a moment here on day 25 to sincerely thank you for giving this a try. You have only a few more days in this program and I really appreciate you trusting me to take you through this. It really does mean a lot to me. I hope you'll continue to be a part of the 90/10 family.

SCHEDULE

Upon Waking: 12-16 oz pure water

Breakfast: Coconut Berry Smoothie (see page 103). We've got a throwback to week 1 on the menu for breakfast.

Midmorning: Drink water throughout the morning. Snack is optional depending on your schedule and if you are truly hungry.

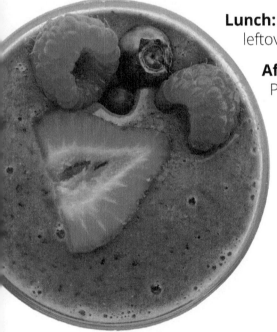

Lunch: Leftover Pork Fried Rice. This is your second leftover serving of this recipe.

Afternoon: Drink water throughout the afternoon. Pick one snack from the options on page 181.

Dinner: One Pan Salmon and Broccoli (see page 121). I guess it's throwback day. Everyone in the test group loved this recipe so much that I decided to put it in again in week 4.

One of my favorite quotes comes from Teddy Roosevelt and I first heard it from author Brene Brown. It goes like this:

"It is not the critic who counts; not the man who points out how the strong man stumbles, or where the doer of deeds could have done them better. The credit belongs to the man who is actually in the arena, whose face is marred by dust and sweat and blood; who strives valiantly; who errs, who comes short again and again, because there is no effort without error and shortcoming; but who does actually strive to do the deeds; who knows great enthusiasms, the great devotions; who spends himself in a worthy cause; who at the best knows in the end the triumph of high achievement, and who at the worst, if he fails, at least fails while daring greatly, so that his place shall never be with those cold and timid souls who neither know victory nor defeat."

In other words, the credit belongs to YOU. The person that is here on day 26 doing the thing. Even if you stumbled along the way, you dared to do, and that credit belongs to you. Finish strong these last few days!

SCHEDULE

Upon Waking: 12-16 oz pure water

Breakfast: Almond Milk Hot Oatmeal. See page 105 for instructions if you need them.

Midmorning: Drink water throughout the morning. Snack is optional depending on your schedule and if you are truly hungry.

Lunch: Leftover White Chicken Chili.

Afternoon: Drink water throughout the afternoon. Pick one snack from the options on page 181.

Dinner: Lettuce Wrapped Carnitas Tacos (see page 165).

NOTE: You'll save half of the carnitas to use as a salad topping at lunch tomorrow.

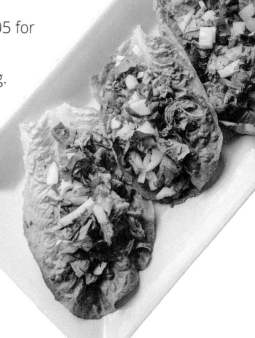

By now, you have nearly 4 weeks of worksheets filled out to look back on. You should be able to see how your actions are related to your energy and how you feel. So, do you need to keep tracking that stuff after the program? Well, you certainly aren't required to. I don't track all of that stuff on a daily basis, but I do use it to self-evaluate when I'm feeling low energy and run down. So, at least keep it in mind as you go forward.

SCHEDULE

Upon Waking: 12-16 oz pure water

Breakfast: Coconut Flour Pancakes with Berries and Maple Syrup (see page 109).

Midmorning: Drink water throughout the morning. Snack is optional depending on your schedule and if you are truly hungry.

Lunch: Mixed Green Salad (see page 113) with leftover carnitas and choice of dressing. Just top your salad with your leftover carnitas from last night.

Afternoon: Drink water throughout the afternoon. Pick one snack from the options on page 181.

Dinner: Thai Chicken Soup (see page 166). This simple soup is big on flavor, but not on prep time.

NOTE: The recipe makes 2 servings, so you'll have one for lunch tomorrow.

Celebration! It's the last day. Congratulations on making it to day 28. You are amazing. Finish strong today and make sure to read the transition section so you have a plan.

SCHEDULE

Upon Waking: 12-16 oz pure water

Breakfast: Coconut Berry Smoothie (see page 103).

Midmorning: Drink water throughout the morning. Snack is optional depending on your schedule and if you are truly hungry.

Lunch: Leftover Thai Chicken Soup

Afternoon: Drink water throughout the afternoon. Pick one snack from the options on page 181.

Dinner: One Pan Pork and Veggies (see page 169). We're finishing this plan off with a beautiful sheet pan meal.

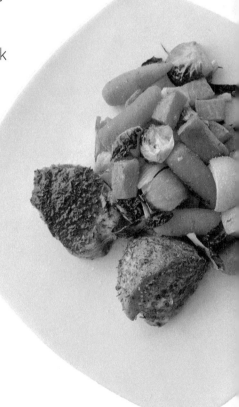

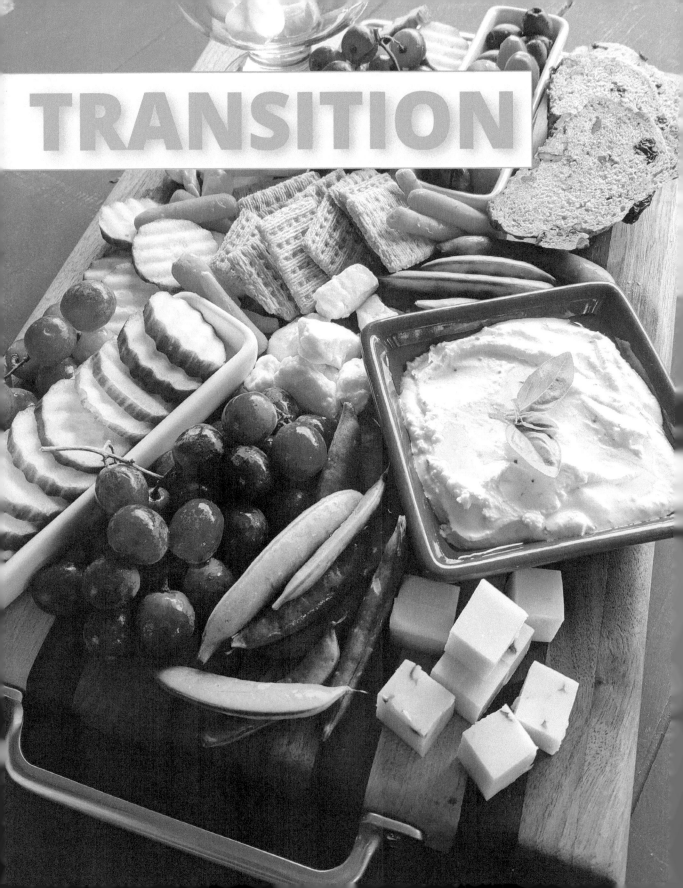

TRANSITION

When you're reading this, you should be in your last week of this 28-day program. Of course, a few of you are reading this before you even start, and that's fine too, but most of you are reading or re-reading this in that last week.

So, you're almost done with a program that is completely laid out for you. For the last 4 weeks, there has been very little guess work. Very little choice. You've been following the plan.

end of this section, I want you to feel excited and confident rather than overwhelmed.

The success of this section is going to depend highly on you taking the advice seriously. My hope is that the way you feel after these last 4 weeks of following the plan will be the motivation you need to keep from eating junk food immediately on day 29. I hope that the benefits you saw from this program will make you take this transition seriously so you

> 66
> ## *Contrary to popular belief, not all celebration has to involve unhealthy food.*
> 99

Now, that's not to say that following a plan is no big deal. *It is* a big deal and we'll celebrate that. But, moving from a set plan to clean eating on your own can be overwhelming and daunting. Of course, it can also be freeing and exciting. It depends on how you look at it and the strategy with which you tackle the task. Perspective is powerful.

My aim in this section is to give you a detailed strategy for transitioning from this set plan to eating clean the 90/10 way on your own. At the

can transform a 28-day success into a lifestyle that will serve you well for years to come.

TRANSITION STEP 1

Evaluation and Celebration: The very first thing you need to do after completing this program is "evaluate and celebrate". Literally, I want you to tally up all the things that went well during the last 28 days and then celebrate them.

This doesn't mean that you need to go out for cheesecake. Contrary to popular belief, not all celebration has to involve unhealthy food. Although, in general, I'm not against celebrating something with a cake, a beer, a margarita, or ice cream, celebrating your 28 days of healthy eating with one of those is a bit counterproductive.

The most important part of this is going to be fairly evaluating your "wins" during this program. Most often, we tend to focus on the negative. If we wanted to lose 10 pounds but we only lost 5, we'll put that in the "loss" column rather than the "win" column. If we stayed on plan 20 out of 28 days, many will call that a failure. Yet, when we exceed goals we tend to minimize that and say it's not that big of a deal.

I want you to do something a bit different. I want you to do your best to find every little tiny thing that could be called a "win". The 5 pounds is a win. If you made dinner at home 20 out of 28 days even if you completely blew it on pizza and ice cream the other 8, those 20 go in the "win" column. Every night you didn't have your normal 2 glasses of wine is a win. Every day you got better sleep is a win. Every bit of energy you felt is a win. Be detailed!

Write the wins down and tell your story of the last 28 days. You don't have to share it with anyone, but write it down anyway. Tell yourself how proud you are of yourself (yes, talk to yourself kindly) in that story.

Now, celebrate it without using junk food. Celebrate the wins. There are a number of ways you could do this from things that cost money to completely free things. You could go shopping, get a massage, go on a quick weekend getaway, have lunch with a friend and share your excitement, share your story on social media so others can celebrate with you, get someone to watch the kids for a night and go to a movie, sign up for a big event, or anything else that feels like celebration to you.

TRANSITION STEP 2

Consider Reintroducing Gluten and Dairy: There is no requirement to ever eat dairy or gluten again. You can get all of the nutrients in these items from other sources, and hopefully you've shown yourself over the course of the last 4 weeks that it's not really that hard to live without them.

With that said, if they don't cause digestive issues, allergic reactions, bloating, or any other negative symptoms, and you want to reintroduce them to your diet, you can. I just recommend that you introduce them one at a time and very slowly so you can be SURE that they aren't causing any issues. I actually still eat gluten and dairy as of this writing, but only because I have cut them out multiple times and reintroduced them systematically wihtout any noticeable issues.

It's important that you don't change too much at once, so here's a sample schedule for reincorporating dairy and wheat:

- **DAY 1:** Have a little non-cultured dairy about 3 times during the day. For example, use whole

whole grain types that meet the green tier requirements. Maybe a slice of 100% whole grain toast with your scramble at breakfast, a 100% whole wheat wrap at lunch, and some pasta at dinner. Again, pay close attention to how you feel. Digestive issues are definitely a concern here, but also be conscious of mood swings, energy levels, and cravings that can be the result of unstable blood sugar and insulin levels.

> **"**
> ## It's important that you don't change too much at once...
> **"**

milk in your oatmeal instead of almond milk, have some cheddar on your lunch salad, and maybe some cheese and sour cream on your chili at dinner. Be conscious of how you feel throughout the day. Look for digestive issues especially.

- **DAYS 2-4:** Go back to dairy free and see if anything changes.

- **DAY 5:** Have some gluten about 3 times during the day but not huge amounts. Keep it to 100%

- **DAYS 6-8:** Go back to gluten free and see if anything changes.

You're welcome to make your own decision about gluten and dairy after you've done your testing. Or, if you'd just prefer to leave them out or severely limit them, you can do that instead.

TRANSITION STEP 3

Go 90/10 Clean: From here, it's time to just eat 90/10 clean. That means you eat 90% of your intake from the green tier, 10% from the yellow tier, and 0% from the red tier (except special occasions). Use PART I of this book to learn it, or use the academy as mentioned below.

You'll become a master of reading ingredient labels and knowing where things are on the tiers. It won't take long at all for clean eating to become nearly second nature to you. You'll spot a processed food with its bogus health claims from a mile away and steer your cart toward the real food.

I have everything all set up to make 90/10 eating as easy as possible. In fact, many (if not all) of the recipes from this book are available on the 90/10 website along with 900+ other recipes that meet the clean eating criteria.

Here are some ideas for how you can easily transition to 90/10 eating:

- **FREE:** Simply go to the main 90/10 website at www.9010nutrition.com and click on the Academy under the "Learn 90/10" menu. Then, go through the simple 90/10 Academy. You can register for a free account and do the entire training in just an hour or so. Then, use the hundreds of recipes on the website as well as any other recipes you find on the web that meet the criteria to create a weekly meal

plan for yourself. If you learn the principles and then plan ahead, you'll be doing just like you did on this plan!

- **MEMBERSHIP:** If you'd like some help with the planning, we do that. Every week, we put out meal plans for our members. Membership is inexpensive and gives you access to 4 different weekly meal plans and a drag-and-drop meal planner. You can literally take one of the meal plans, copy it to your drag and drop meal planner, modify it to your tastes and preferences, and then generate a shopping list with a few clicks. You can try it free for 3 weeks at www.9010nutrition.com/learn-more. This is a great way to just keep right on going with your new lifestyle.

As you stick with a 90/10 lifestyle, you'll learn how to use freezer meals, a slow cooker, an Instant Pot, the meal planner, "1-2-3 Eat!" principles, sheet pan meals, and more. You'll be able to throw together a 28-day plan just like this all by yourself!

Make sure to give yourself the time to learn. You can't expect to go straight from this 28-day plan into doing it yourself with no bumps. You need to learn through doing. So DO! I'll be there with you the whole time (see the next step).

TRANSITION STEP 4

Become a Part of The Community: If you haven't joined our Facebook community, this is a great time. You'll get the support of or at your local coffee shop. That's up to you. But, there are millions of people out there struggling with food. They're starving themselves on low calorie diets, drinking canned meal replacement shakes, and maybe even doing the cabbage soup diet. You can tell them about something different.

> " **You need to learn through doing. So DO!** "

seasoned veterans of 90/10 as well as new people. You can find a link to the group right on the homepage at www.9010nutrition.com.

TRANSITION STEP 5

Share Your Story: If you had a great experience with this program, I encourage you to share that with others. You can do it through Facebook, Instagram, Pinterest, email,

If you'd like to recommend the program, just send them to 28daystoclean.com and hashtag #28daystoclean.

I'd also be so thrilled to hear your stories. So, if you write up your story, be sure to send it to ryan@9010nutrition.com and let me know if you're ok with me sharing it. I'll feature many of them on the website and our social channels.

ⓘ REMINDER

You can find helpful additional resources such as printables and links online at www.28daystoclean.com/resources (or simply use the QR code to the right).

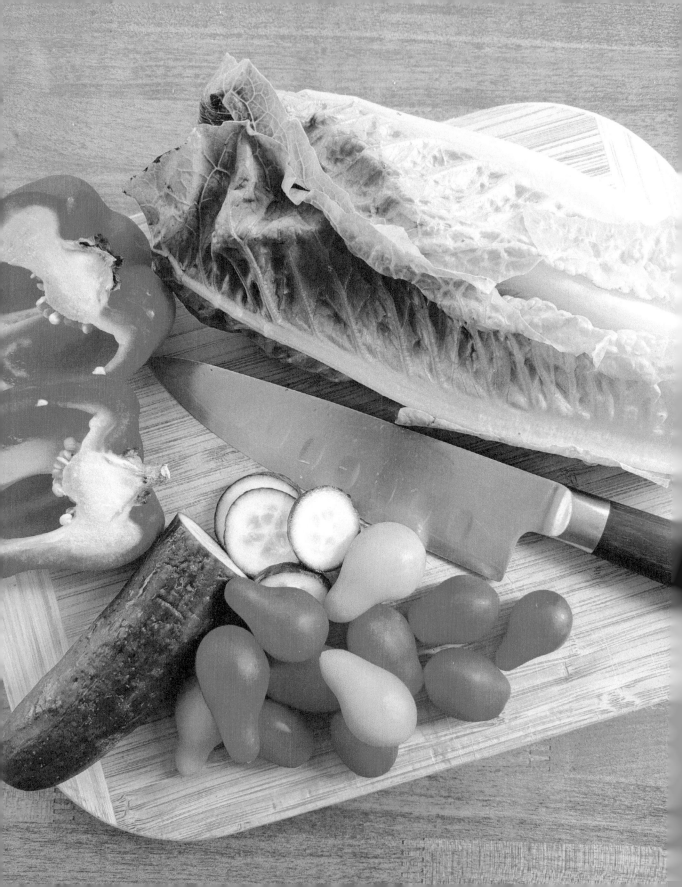

PART III
THE RECIPES

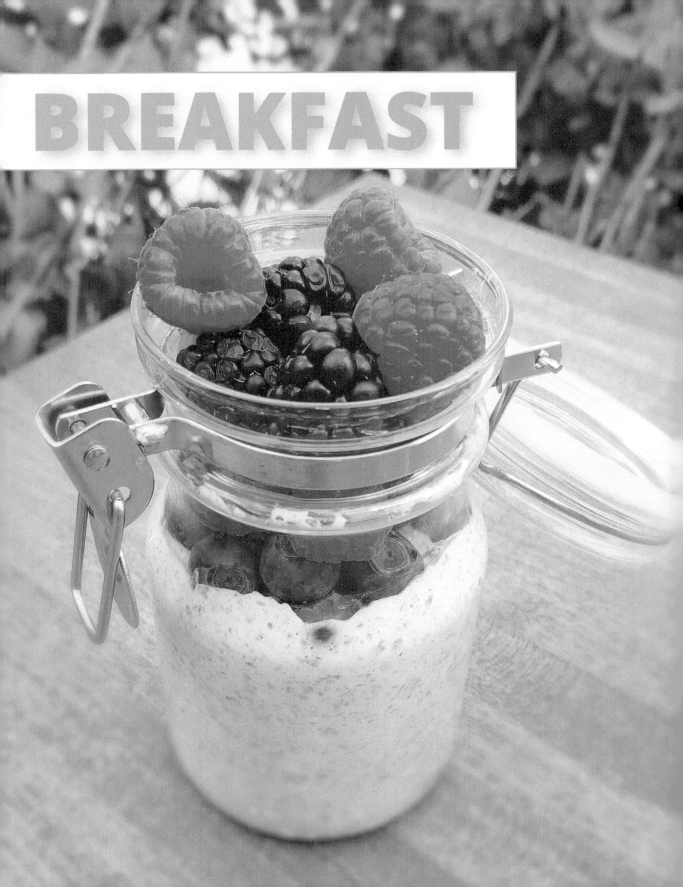

BREAKFAST

These simple but tasty breakfast recipes are intended to give you the perfect mix of variety and familiarity. There should be just enough repeating to make it doable but enough variety to keep it from being boring. This is exactly how I love to eat.

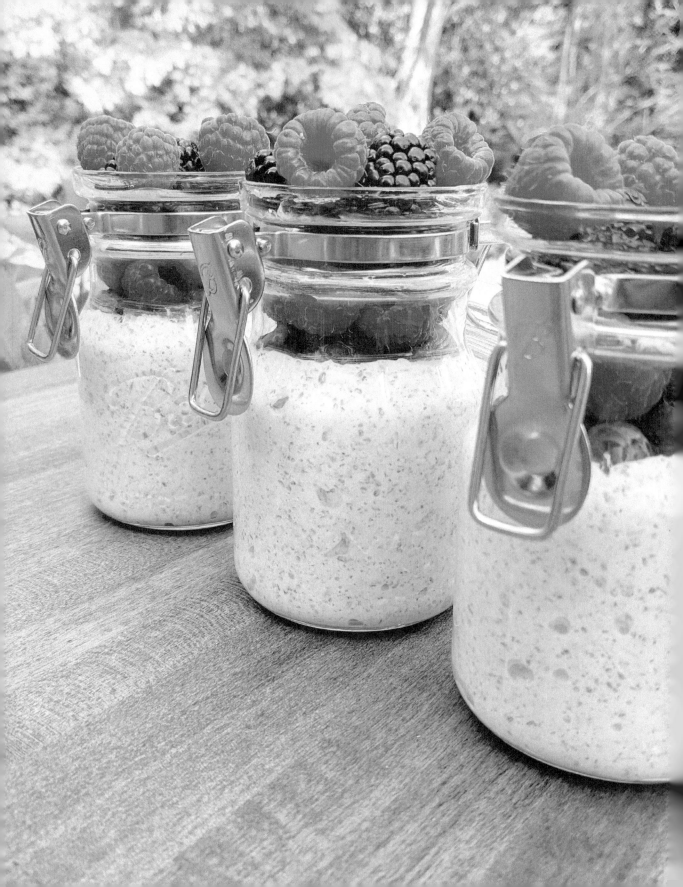

OVERNIGHT OATS

Servings: 3 | Prep Time: 10 min | Cook Time: Overnight

You'll be making overnight oats during the prep section for some weeks. These will be super easy, grab-and-go breakfasts.

You can use these in place of the hot oatmeal later in the program if you like them better as well.

2 cups old fashioned rolled oats (gluten free)

1 cup Greek or regular yogurt (plain, unsweetened)

1 1/2 cups unsweetened almond milk

3 Tbsp flax meal or chia seeds

2 cups fresh or frozen berries of choice

honey for sweetener

1. Mix the oats, yogurt, almond milk, and chia/flax in a large bowl. Let stand for 30 minutes.

2. Divide the oatmeal mixture into three mason jars or resealable containers. Add fruit toppings.

3. Seal and place in the fridge overnight and up to 1 week.

4. When ready to eat, drizzle some honey for sweetener (optional) and enjoy.

3-EGG SCRAMBLE OR OMELET

Servings: 1 | Prep Time: 5 min | Cook Time: 10 min

You can either make this as a scramble or as an omelet. The power of egg protein, veggies, and avocado in the morning is a thing of beauty. I suggest topping this with some Cholula hot sauce, but a fresh salsa or just as is works fine too.

3 eggs

1/4 red bell pepper, diced

1/2 cup spinach, fresh (or kale or other green leafy vegetable)

1/4 onion small, diced

1 Tbsp extra virgin olive oil (or butter, avocado oil, or coconut oil)

1/2 haas avocado, small

1. Dice the onion and bell pepper. Add oil or butter to a medium skillet and heat to medium high. Add the veggies and cook for 2-3 minutes or until they begin to soften.

2. Beat the eggs well.

3. Add the spinach and then pour the eggs over the veggies and stir and chop with a spatula until the eggs dry out or let the bottom dry out and fold in half to make an omelet.

4. Top with diced avocado and serve with your favorite hot sauce if desired.

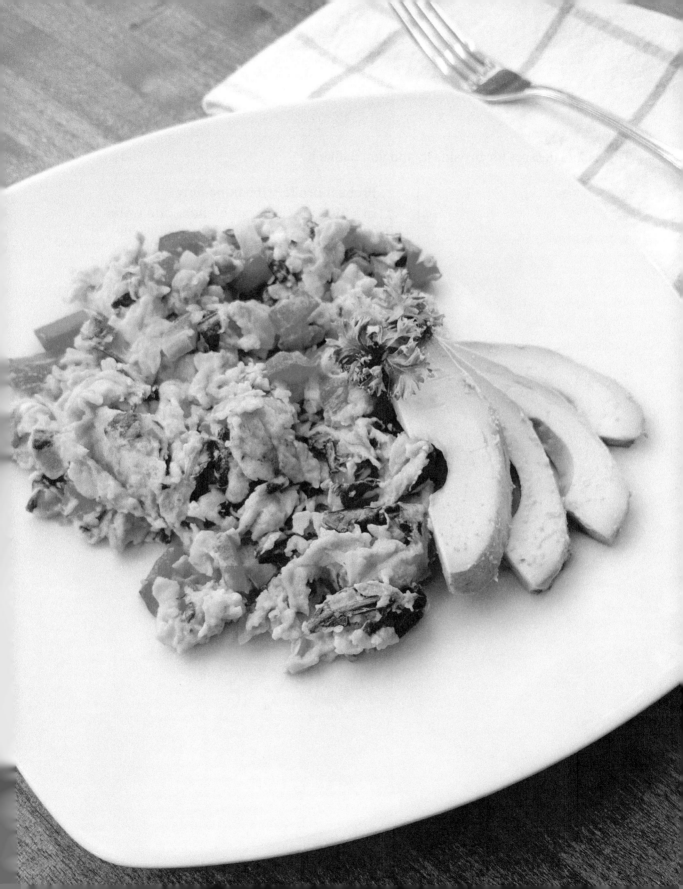

BREAKFAST BERRY CRISP

Servings: 3 | Prep Time: 15 min | Cook Time: 15 min

This is like dessert for breakfast, and you'll love it.

1/2 cup walnuts

1/2 cup pecans

1/4 teaspoon cinnamon

1/8 teaspoon cardamom or nutmeg

1 Tbsp unsalted butter, cut into small pieces

1 tsp vanilla

3 cups berries (fresh or frozen)

1 Tbsp honey (optional)

1 1/2 cup Greek or regular yogurt (plain, unsweetened)

1. Preheat broiler (if baking now).

2. In a food processor or blender, add walnuts, pecans, cinnamon, cardamom/nutmeg and butter and pulse a few times until everything is just mixed.

3. In a small pot, heat berries with vanilla and honey. Bring to a gentle boil for 5 minutes, so the berries are well heated. Drain off most of the liquid.

4. Spoon the berry mixture into 3 ramekins or into one baking dish.

5. Spoon the nut mixture evenly on top of the berries.

6. If baking now, put under the broiler and heat for 3-5 minutes until the topping is lightly browned. Take care not to let the topping burn under the broiler.

7. If you plan on baking individual servings each morning, just wrap the individual ramekins with foil and place in the fridge. When ready to eat, bake at 350 for about 12 minutes until it is heated through. You can turn it to broiler and crisp the top if you wish but that is optional.

8. Serve with 1/2 cup Greek or plain yogurt.

COCONUT BERRY SMOOTHIE

Servings: 1 | Prep Time: 5 min | Cook Time: N/A

This smoothie makes a great, quick breakfast in the blender. It's easy and healthy with good fats that help keep you full and full of energy.

This recipe doesn't include any sweetener. I recommend you give it a try as is and then add a bit of honey if you really want it a bit sweeter.

1/2 cup coconut milk (canned unsweetened, full fat)

1 cup unsweetened almond milk

1 cup frozen berries (blueberries, raspberries, strawberries, etc.)

1 Tbsp almond butter

1/2 cup water

1. Combine ingredients in a blender. Blend and enjoy.

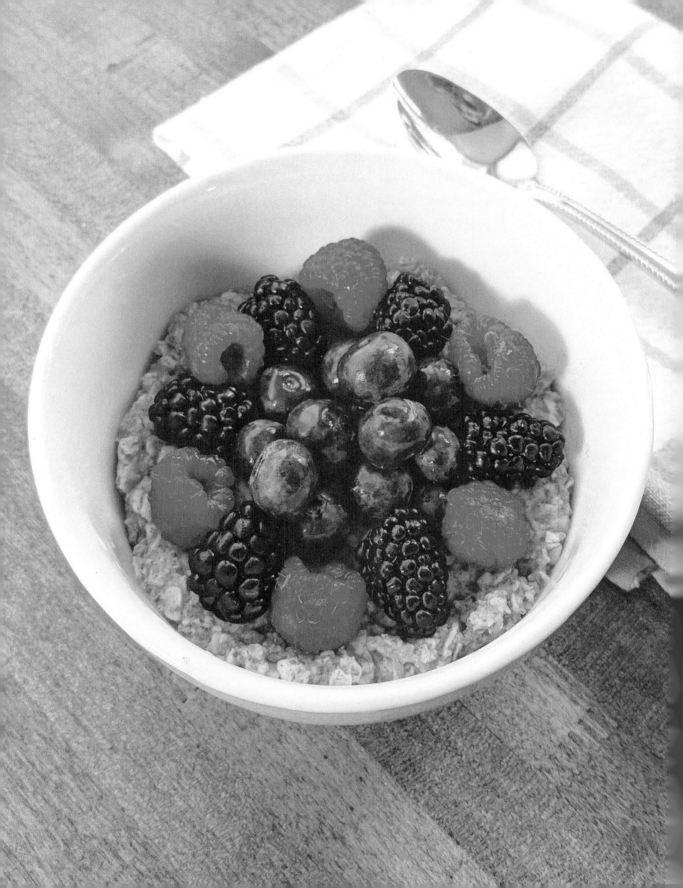

ALMOND MILK HOT OATMEAL

Servings: 3 | Prep Time: 10 min | Cook Time: 10 min

This hot oatmeal recipe comes out so colorful with fresh or even frozen berries. If you follow the weekly prep instructions, you'll save some time by making up packets of the dry ingredients at the beginning of the week. Then, you can just heat it up with the almond milk and serve!

Dry Ingredients

2 cups rolled oats (gluten free)

1/4 cup walnuts

3 Tbsp flax meal or chia seeds

1 tsp cinnamon

Wet Ingredients

2 1/4 cups unsweetened almond milk

2 cups fresh or frozen berries of choice

honey for sweetener

1. Add 1 cup of oats and all of the walnuts to a blender or food processor and pulse until powdery.

2. Add the blender contents, the rest of the oats, the flax, and the cinnamon to a large bowl and mix well.

3. Divide the oatmeal mixture into three resealable baggies or containers.

4. On the morning you are going to eat a serving, add ¾ cup of almond milk and one bag of the dry mix to a small saucepan.

5. Heat over medium heat until the mixture begins to thicken (about 5 minutes). Add the berries and honey and serve.

6. NOTE: The hot oatmeal seems to do a good job of thawing the berries (if using frozen berries). They are a nice temperature when mixed, in my opinion. If you find that they are still frozen or you don't like the feeling of cold berries in hot oatmeal, you can heat them with the mixture in the saucepan or use fresh berries.

BACON AND EGG MUFFINS

Servings: 3 | Prep Time: 10 min | Cook Time: 20 min

These are great to make ahead of time and reheat when you are ready to eat them. Of course, you can also make them on demand if you wish. Silicone muffin cups are amazing for these, but a greased muffin tin will work just fine.

6 oz uncured bacon (no sugar listed in ingredients, such as Hempler's)

8 eggs

1/2 tsp salt

1/2 tsp pepper

extra virgin olive oil or coconut oil, for greasing the pan

1/2 red bell pepper, finely diced (or other veggies)

1. Cook the bacon first (any way you like). You can cook it in the oven or on a griddle or a pan on the stove. Example: Preheat oven to 400 F. Line a baking sheet with parchment paper. Lay bacon slices on parchment, trying not to let them touch. Bake at 400 F for 20 min. Allow to cool slightly. Crumble.

2. For the muffins, preheat the oven to 350 F.

3. Add eggs, salt, and pepper to a medium bowl. Beat with a whisk until well-beaten.

4. Grease 9 standard (2-3/4") muffin cups/tins with coconut, avocado or olive oil and then divide the egg mixture evenly between all muffin cups.

5. Divide the bacon and red pepper (or other veggies) evenly between the muffins by sprinkling them into the egg mixture.

6. Bake at 350 F for 20 minutes or until eggs are fully set. Divide into 3 servings (3 muffins each).

7. Feel free to add spinach, mushrooms or other veggies as desired.

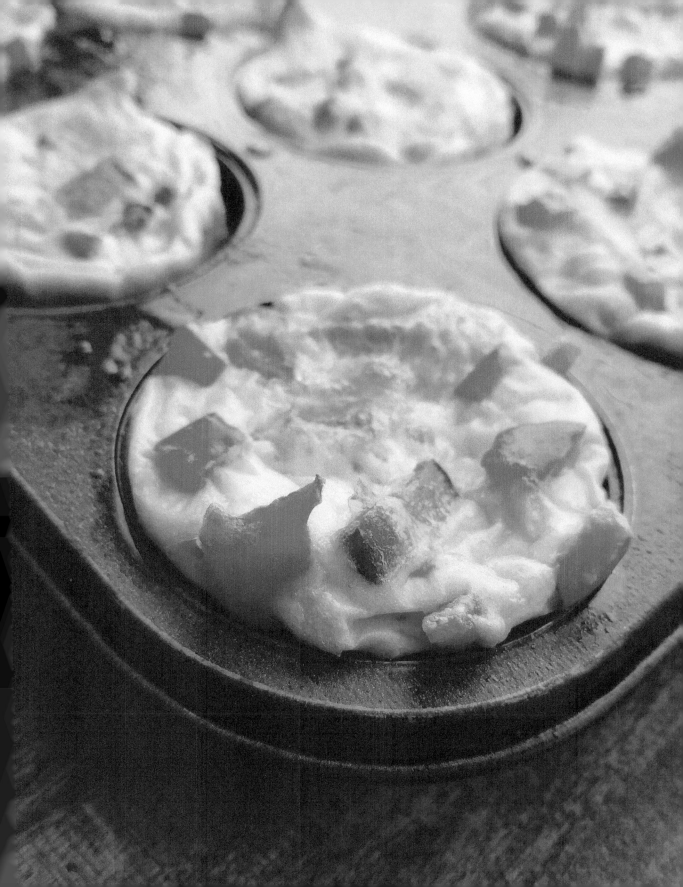

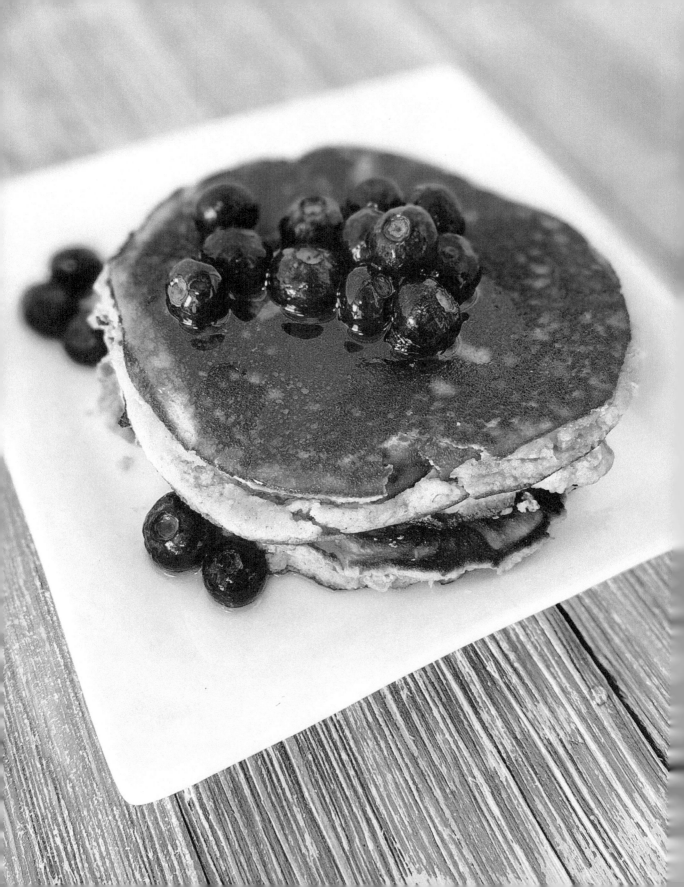

COCONUT FLOUR PANCAKES

Servings: 1 | Prep Time: 10 min | Cook Time: 10 min

The flavor of these pancakes is simply wonderful. However, I will warn you that these take extra care over normal pancakes. It's not extra time, but they are a bit harder to flip and easy to burn if you don't watch them.

1/4 cup coconut flour

1/4 teaspoon baking soda

2 eggs

2 Tbsp almond butter

1 tablespoon honey

1/4 cup unsweetened applesauce

1/4 cup unsweetened almond milk

berries, optional

pure maple syrup, optional

butter for cooking

1. Mix the coconut flour and baking soda together in a small bowl.

2. In a larger bowl, beat the 2 eggs. Then add the almond butter, honey, applesauce, and almond milk and stir until well mixed.

3. Add the coconut flour mix to the wet ingredients and stir until combined. It will be thick to the point that you can pour it but just barely. You can use coconut flour and water to adjust if needed but you should need a spatula to help you "pour" it onto the pan.

4. Add a bit of butter to a pan or griddle and then pour/spoon the pancake batter into 3 pancakes. This batter won't bubble like normal pancake batter, so watch it closely so it doesn't burn on the bottom. Flip it when it is cooked enough on the bottom to get a spatula under it.

5. Cook for 1-2 minutes on the second side and then remove from the pan.

6. Top with berries and maple syrup if desired. Go easy on the syrup because these pancakes are pretty sweet on their own.

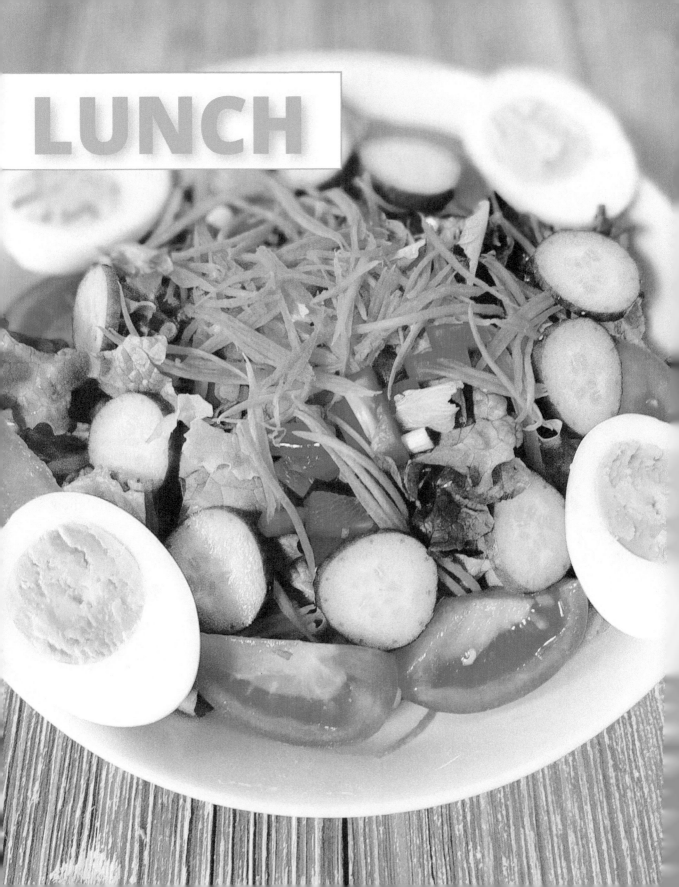

LUNCH

Mixed Green Salad   **113**

The lunch recipes list is a bit short, but have no fear. The reason there aren't a lot of recipes here is that you'll mostly be utilizing intentional leftovers for your lunches. This way, you will rarely need to prepare and cook an additional recipe for lunch.

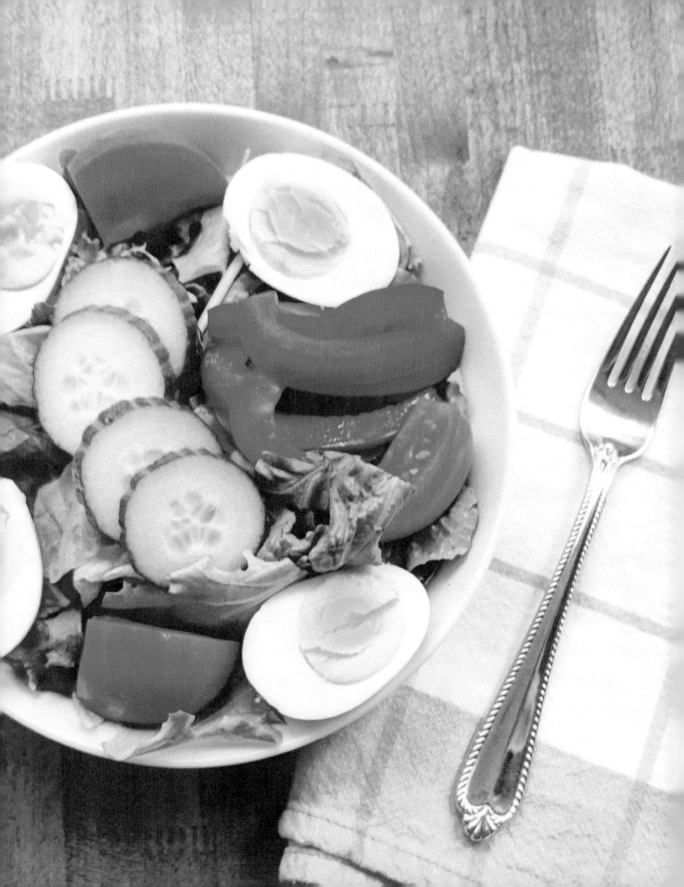

MIXED GREEN SALAD

Servings: 1 | Prep Time: 10 min | Cook Time: N/A

We'll use this salad as a base and add various proteins such as hard-boiled eggs, leftover steak, and leftover chicken. Feel free to use your favorite veggies and healthy green tier salad ingredients. For this plan, stay away from changing the recipe by adding things like cheese or croutons. Different healthy veggies and lettuces are fine.

3 cups mixed salad greens, romaine, or other lettuce

1/2 cup diced veggies (bell pepper, cucumber, tomato, mushrooms, etc.)

1/2 haas avocado, optional

1. Combine into an amazing salad.

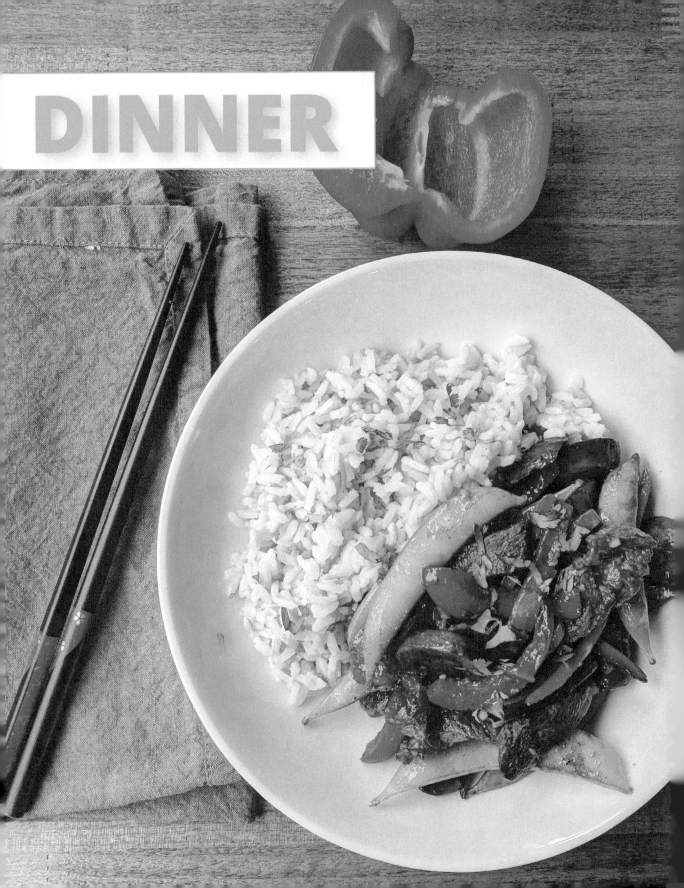

DINNER

The goal with these dinner recipes is to give you tasty and interesting dinners without hard-to-find ingredients, overly-complicated instructions, or long prep and cook times. It seems like a lofty goal, but it really isn't as hard as it sounds.

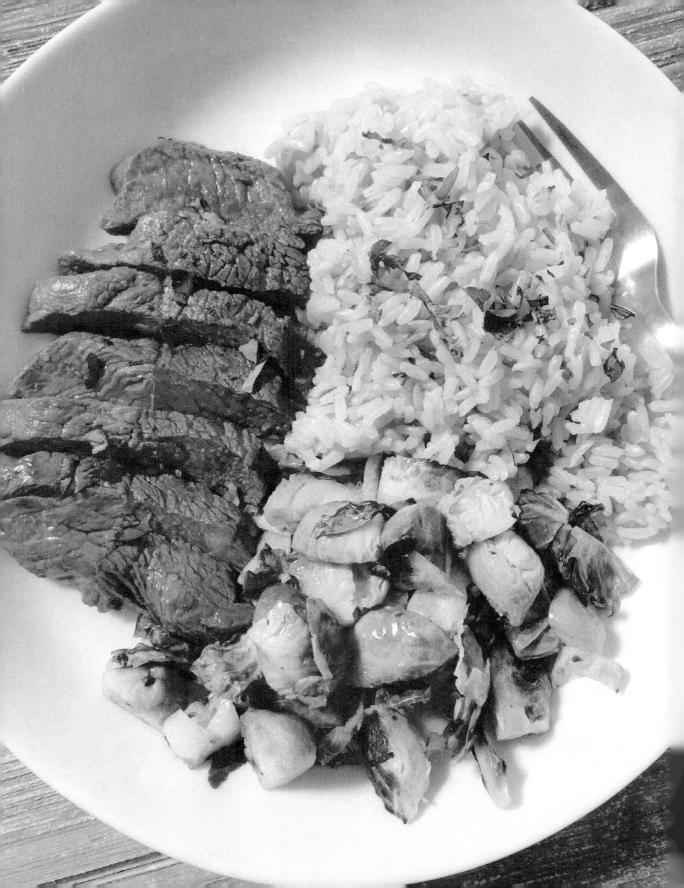

BALSAMIC STEAK WITH BRUSSELS SPROUTS AND BROWN RICE

Servings: 2* | Prep Time: 15 min | Cook Time: 20 min

This recipe is a classic example of a simple "1-2-3 Eat!" meal. It combines a protein (steak), a veggie (Brussels sprouts), and a healthy starch (brown rice). It's simple and effective and the number of different options are nearly endless.

*You're making 2 servings of the steak but not the sides. The second serving of steak will be used as a topping for a lunch salad.

8 oz sirloin steak, grass-fed if possible

1 cup Brussels sprouts, quartered and destemmed

1/4 onion, diced

1 Tbsp bottled minced garlic

1/2 cup brown rice, cooked

butter (optional)

2 Tbsp extra virgin olive oil

2 Tbsp balsamic vinegar

salt

pepper

1. Salt the steak liberally and then add it to a resealable bag along with 1 Tbsp of oil and all of the balsamic vinegar. Refrigerate for at least 20 minutes.

2. Heat the grill to medium-high.

3. Grill the steak to your liking.

4. Heat the remaining olive oil in a skillet and add the onion. Sauté until the onion softens (3 minutes).

5. Add the garlic and Brussels sprouts to the pan, salt and pepper liberally, and cook until the edges of the brussels sprouts begin to brown. They should still be firm.

6. Serve half of the steak (4 oz), with ½ cup of cooked brown rice (see prep section of week 1), and all of the Brussels. You can add butter and salt to the rice if you wish.

7. Slice the other half of the steak and save for tomorrow's lunch.

CHICKEN AND BROWN RICE

Servings: 3 | Prep Time: 15 min | Cook Time: 20 min+

This one can be done in the Instant Pot or the stove top. I prefer the Instant Pot because it's just so easy. I've also tried making this in the slow cooker, but it doesn't save a lot of time because the rice has to be added later.

You're making 3 servings of this with this recipe. The other two will be for lunches.

1 Tbsp unsalted butter

1/2 onion small, chopped

1 carrot large, chopped

1/2 cup mushrooms, sliced

1 Tbsp bottled minced garlic

1 cup brown rice, uncooked

1 Tbsp Italian seasoning

1/4 tsp salt

1/8 tsp pepper

1 cup chicken broth

8 oz boneless, skinless chicken breasts

1/2 cup frozen green peas

fresh parsley, optional garnish

Instant Pot

1. Press "sauté" on the Instant Pot. Add the butter to melt. Add onion, garlic and carrot. Sauté 3-5 min.

2. Add brown rice, Italian seasoning, salt, and pepper. Sauté for 3 minutes. Push "cancel".

3. Add chicken broth, mix well, and scrape bottom and edges of the insert so all of the rice and veggies are in the liquid. Add chicken on top of the rice mixture. Do not mix. Close the Instant Pot lid and set the valve to "sealing". Program for manual-high and 20 minutes.

4. Allow for 10 min natural pressure release, then carefully vent the rest of the pressure.

5. Remove the lid and move the chicken to a cutting board. Add mushrooms and frozen peas to the rice mixture in the Instant Pot and stir well.

6. Put the lid back on the Instant Pot and move the valve to sealing. Leave sealed but not on for 5 minutes and then release pressure.

7. Chop chicken or shred with 2 forks. Add chicken back to the pot and mix well. Serve in bowls with fresh parsley.

Stove Top

1. Add butter to a large saucepan over medium-high heat. Add chopped onion, garlic and carrot. Sauté 3-5 minutes. Meanwhile, dice the chicken into ½ inch pieces.

2. Add Italian seasoning, salt, and pepper and continue to sauté for another 3 minutes.

3. Add chicken broth. Mix well. Add diced chicken and bring to a boil. Boil 5-7 minutes or until the chicken is cooked through.

4. Reduce heat to low, add rice, peas, and mushrooms, and cook for 60 minutes or until the rice is tender. Serve in bowls with fresh parsley.

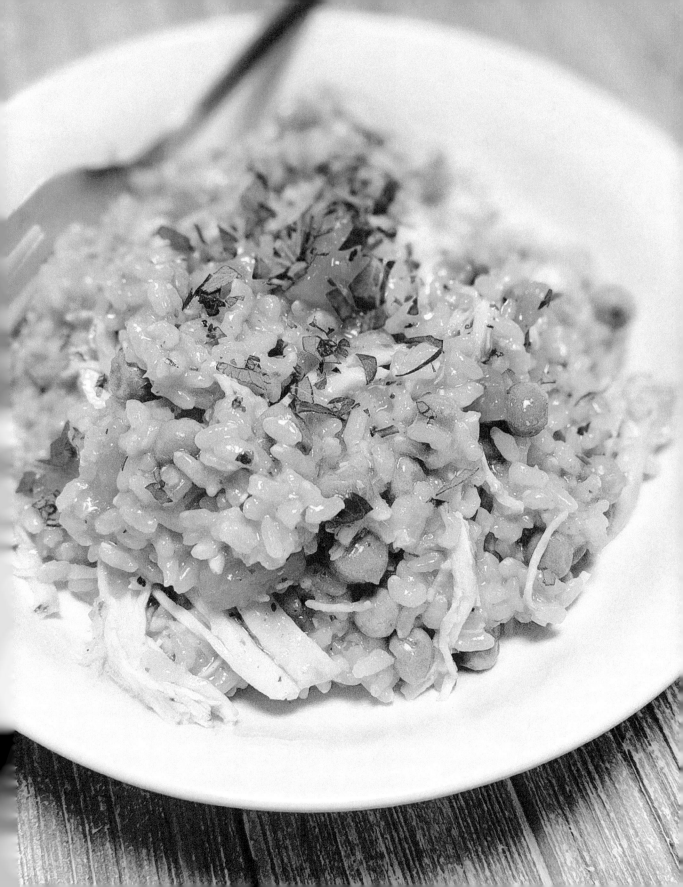

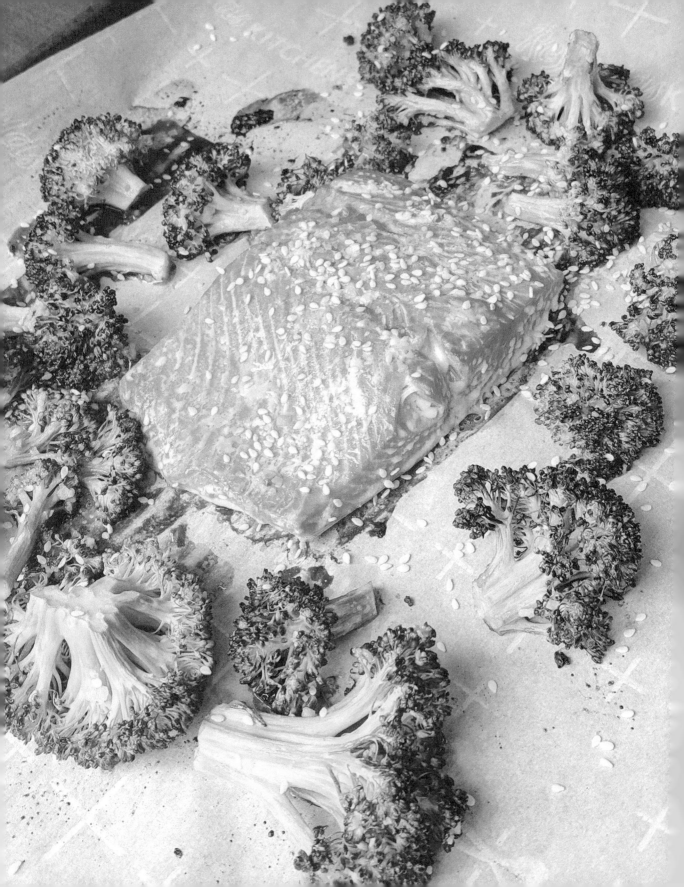

ONE PAN SALMON AND BROCCOLI

Servings: 1 | Prep Time: 5 min | Cook Time: 15 min

This one pan salmon and broccoli dinner will surprise you just like it did the test group. It's so simple but oh so tasty. Plus, just like with any one pan meal, clean up is a breeze.

One test group participant said: *"This Salmon and Broccoli dinner was great! My husband loved it too. First thing he said after the first bite was "yummmmmm". Wonderful recipe for this lovely little piece of fresh, wild caught Sockeye Salmon."*

1 salmon fillet, 4-6 oz

2 Tbsp sesame oil, divided

2 Tbsp Bragg Liquid Aminos, divided

2 green onions, thinly sliced

2 tsp sesame seeds

2 cups broccoli florets

1 Tbsp bottled minced garlic

1 Tbsp coconut oil, melted

1. Preheat oven to 400 F. Combine broccoli, garlic, and half of the sesame oil and all of the coconut oil in a large bowl. Toss to coat.

2. Arrange salmon on a parchment-lined baking sheet. Drizzle with about half of the sesame oil and liquid aminos.

3. Arrange the broccoli in a single layer around the salmon.

4. Bake at 400 F for 15 minutes or until broccoli is beginning to brown and fish flakes easily with a fork.

5. Remove from oven, and return the broccoli to bowl. Add Bragg Liquid Aminos. Toss well. Place in serving dish. Top with sesame seeds.

6. Sprinkle the onions and sesame seeds on the salmon. Serve.

STEAK FAJITA ROLLUPS WITH GREEN BEANS

Servings: 2* | Prep Time: 15 min | Cook Time: 20 min

These rollups are so fun and colorful, you won't miss the tortilla. Also, if you don't know, 7-minute green beans are famous in the 90/10 world. You have to cook them for exactly 7 minutes (unless you really like to give me a hard time...then you cook them for 7 "ish" minutes).

*You're making 2 servings of the rollups but not the green beans. The second serving of steak rollups will be used as a topping for a lunch salad.

1/4 onion, large, cut into strips

1 bell pepper cut into strips, any color or combo

1 lb skirt steak or flank steak

1/2 Tbsp chili powder

1/2 Tbsp cumin

1/2 tsp onion powder

1/2 tsp garlic powder

1/4 tsp oregano

1/4 tsp paprika

1/4 tsp salt

1/4 tsp pepper

1 Tbsp extra virgin olive oil

1/2 lb green beans, trimmed

butter (optional)

1. Mix all the spices (chili powder through pepper) in a small bowl.

2. Add pepper and onion strips to a large ziploc bag (or a large bowl). Add olive oil and half of the spice mix to the bag or bowl and mix well.

3. Over medium heat in a grill pan or frying pan, cook the peppers and onions until desired tenderness (or in a veggie basket on grill).

4. Cut the beef into thin strips about 4-5 inches long by 2 inches wide. Rub both sides of the beef strips with the remaining spice mix.

5. Roll the onions and peppers into the beef strips and secure with toothpicks.

6. Cook them until all sides are browned in the same grill pan or on the grill (about 2 minutes each side).

7. For the green beans, bring a medium pot of water to a boil. Add green beans. Boil 7 minutes. Drain and serve. Use butter and salt if desired.

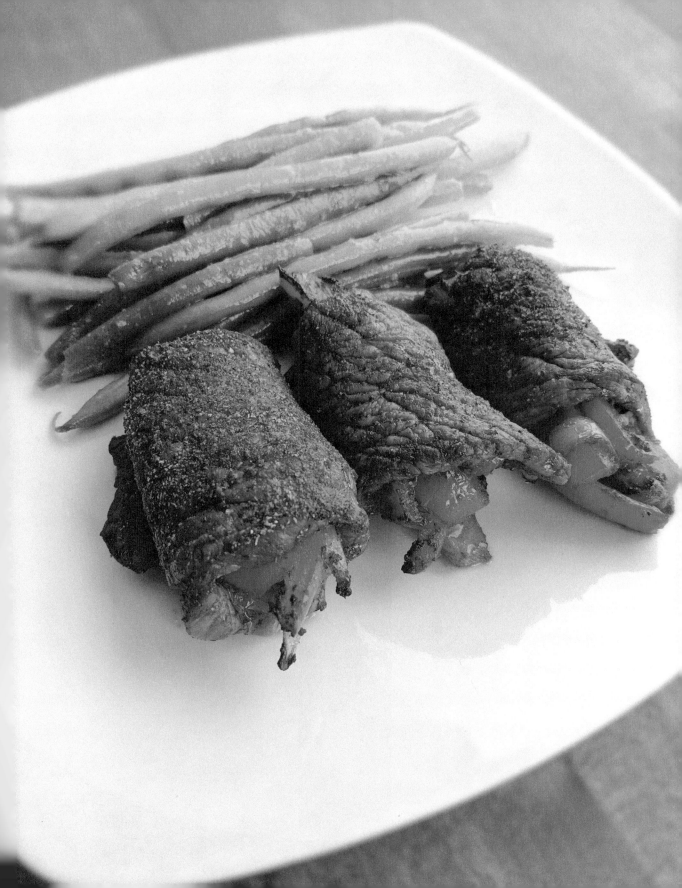

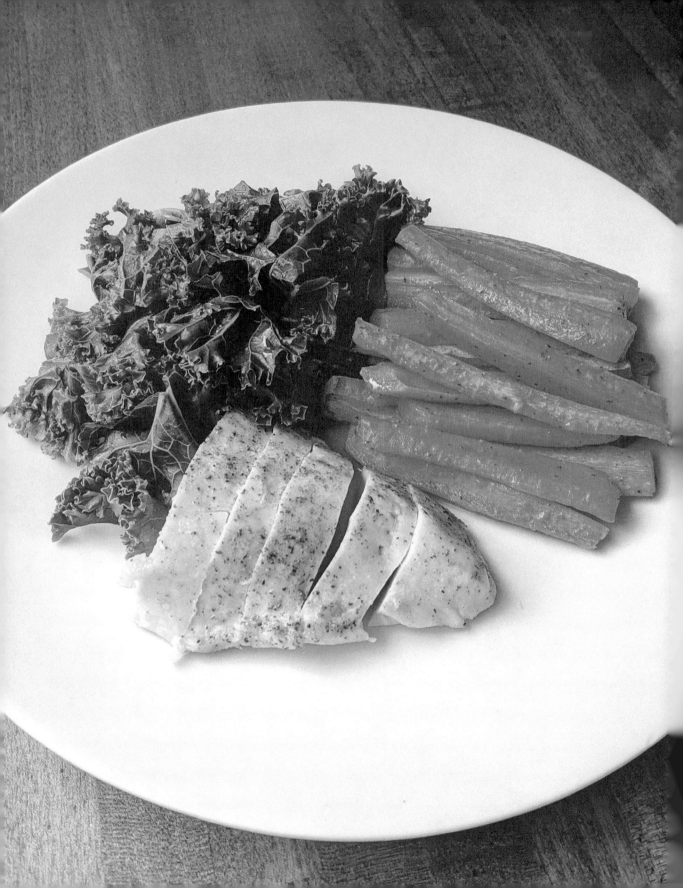

ONE PAN CHICKEN AND CARROT FRIES WITH STEAMED KALE

Servings: 2* | Prep Time: 15 min | Cook Time: 25-30 min

Another one pan dish paired with my wife's absolute favorite thing ever: steamed kale with lemon juice. I know, it's a bit odd, but she would eat it every night. I'll admit that it isn't my favorite (I like many other veggies better), but I like this just fine too. I didn't sell that very well, did I?

*You're making 2 servings of the chicken and carrot fries but not the kale. The second serving of the chicken and fries is for lunch.

10-12 oz boneless, skinless chicken breasts

2 Tbsp extra virgin olive oil, divided

1 lb carrots

salt

pepper

3 cups kale, destemmed and chopped

1 Tbsp lemon juice

1. Preheat oven to 400 F.

2. Peel and cut carrots into wedges.

3. Combine carrots, 1 Tbsp oil, salt and pepper in a bowl or bag. Toss well to coat.

4. Arrange chicken and carrots in a single layer on a parchment-lined baking sheet. Sprinkle chicken with salt, pepper, and any other spices you wish.

5. Bake at 400 F for 30 min or until chicken is done and carrots are tender.

6. To steam the kale, place the kale in a steamer basket over boiling water for 3-5 minutes. Toss with 1 Tbsp olive oil, 1 Tbsp lemon juice, and salt.

7. Save half of the chicken and half of the carrots for lunch tomorrow.

TACO RICE BOWLS

Servings: 3 | Prep Time: 15 min | Cook Time: 20 min

Yes! Tacos in a bowl. You're making 3 servings with this recipe. So, be sure to make a couple of leftover packs for lunches.

1 lb ground beef, 90% lean or leaner

1 can black beans, rinsed and drained

2 Tbsp chili powder

2 Tbsp cumin

3/4 tsp garlic powder

3/4 tsp onion powder

3/4 tsp salt

1/4 tsp oregano

1/4 tsp paprika

1/4 tsp pepper

1 1/2 cup brown rice, cooked

1 cup corn, fresh or frozen

1/2 cup salsa, no sugar listed in ingredients

4 oz romaine lettuce, shredded

1/4 cup cilantro, chopped

1 haas avocado, sliced or diced

1. Brown beef in a medium skillet, stirring to break up chunks, 5-8 minutes or until no longer pink.

2. Add black beans, chili powder, cumin, oregano, paprika, garlic powder, onion powder, salt, and pepper along with 1/2 cup water. Stir well.

3. Bring to a simmer and simmer, uncovered, 15 minutes or until sauce is thickened.

4. Heat the corn in a small saucepan in water until warmed through.

5. Assemble three bowls by evenly dividing the ingredients. Start with 1/3 of the rice in each bowl, and top each bowl with lettuce, taco meat and black beans, corn, salsa, cilantro, and avocado.

6. Save 2 of the bowls for lunches.

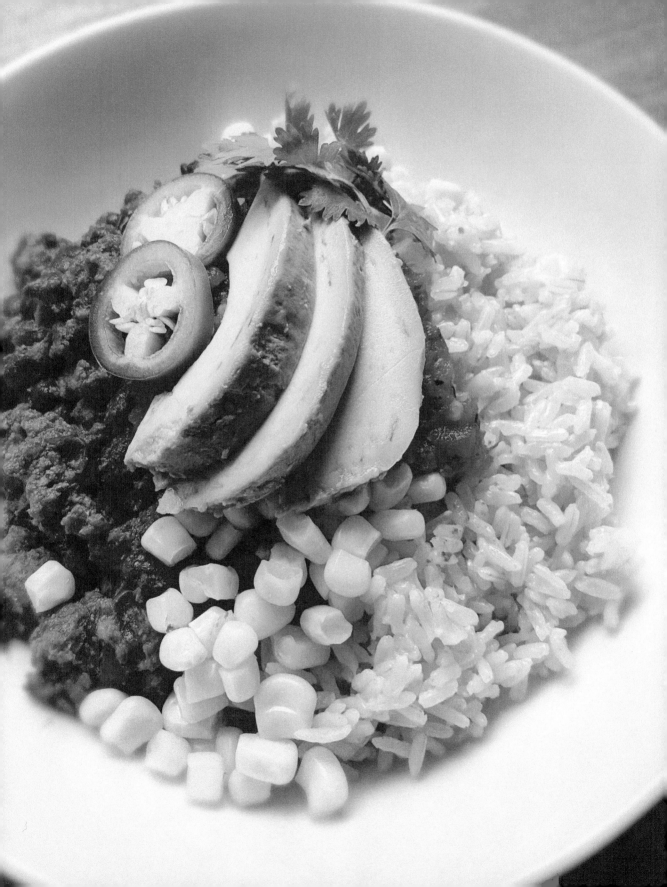

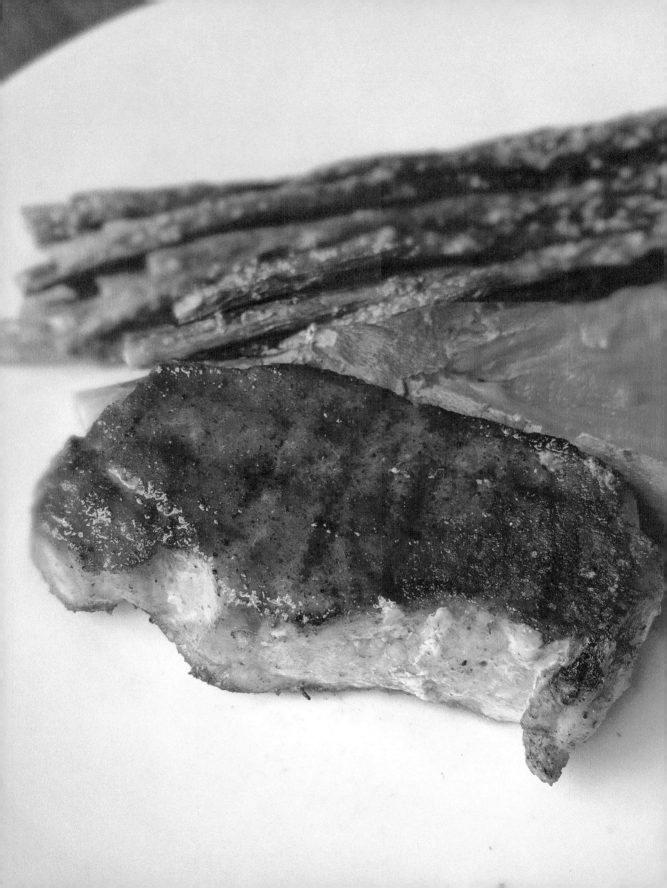

CURRY GRILLED PORK CHOPS WITH SWEET POTATOES AND ASPARAGUS

Servings: 1 | Prep Time: 10 min | Cook Time: 45-60 min

1-2-3 Eat! The curry pork chops are surprisingly simple but flavorful.

1 pork chop bone-in or boneless, 4-6 oz

2 Tbsp extra virgin olive oil, divided

2 tsp curry powder

salt

pepper

1 sweet potato or yam (small, or half of a large)

1 small bunch asparagus, about 4 oz

butter, optional

1. Preheat oven to 400 F. Pierce the sweet potato several times with a knife, wrap in foil, place on a baking sheet, and bake for 1 hour or until tender.

2. Toss asparagus in olive oil, salt and pepper.

3. About 30 minutes before the potato is done, preheat grill to medium.

4. About 15 minutes before potato is done, add asparagus to the baking sheet and bake for the last 15 minutes.

5. Season pork chop with salt and pepper on both sides.

6. Mix remaining olive oil (or about 1 Tbsp) and curry powder in a small bowl and brush both sides of chop with the curry oil mixture.

7. Grill pork chop for 4-6 minutes per side or until done to your liking.

8. NOTE: You may also cook the potato in the Instant Pot or microwave for faster cooking.

RYAN'S BEEF CHILI

Servings: 2 | Prep Time: 15 min | Cook Time: 20 min+

Behold, the highly disputed champion of the chili world. I kid because Heidi and I go back and forth on whose chili is the best, but in all seriousness, this chili is very tasty and healthy at the same time. Perfect.

This recipe makes 2 servings. One will be used as a lunch.

2 cans diced tomatoes, 15 oz

1 can red kidney beans, 15 oz

1/2 yellow onion medium, diced

1/2 bell pepper any color you choose

1/2 lb ground beef, 90% lean or leaner

5-10 slices pickled jalapenos (optional), add more or less to adjust heat

1 Tbsp juice from jalapeno jar

1/2 tsp salt

1 Tbsp chili powder, add more or less to adjust heat

1 tsp extra virgin olive oil

1. Dice onion and bell pepper and sauté in olive oil for 3 minutes over medium heat in a skillet. Remove from skillet.

2. Brown a full pound of ground beef in the same skillet. Drain grease. Reserve half of the ground beef for another recipe and half for this recipe.

3. Combine tomatoes and beans in crock pot or large sauce pan.

4. Add the 1/2 lb of beef, onion, and bell pepper.

5. Add jalapeno slices and jalapeno juice.

6. Add salt and chili powder to taste.

7. Allow to cook on low heat until warmed through. It is now ready to eat, however, it is recommended that you cook it for several hours to allow the flavors to mingle. I usually put it in the crockpot in the morning and have it for dinner that evening.

8. Reserve half of this recipe for use as a lunch.

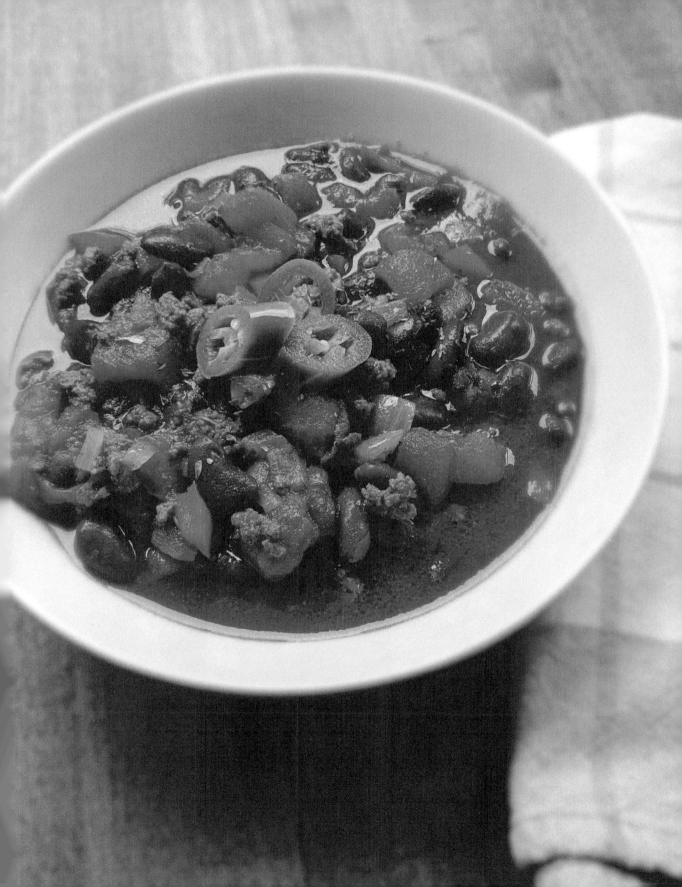

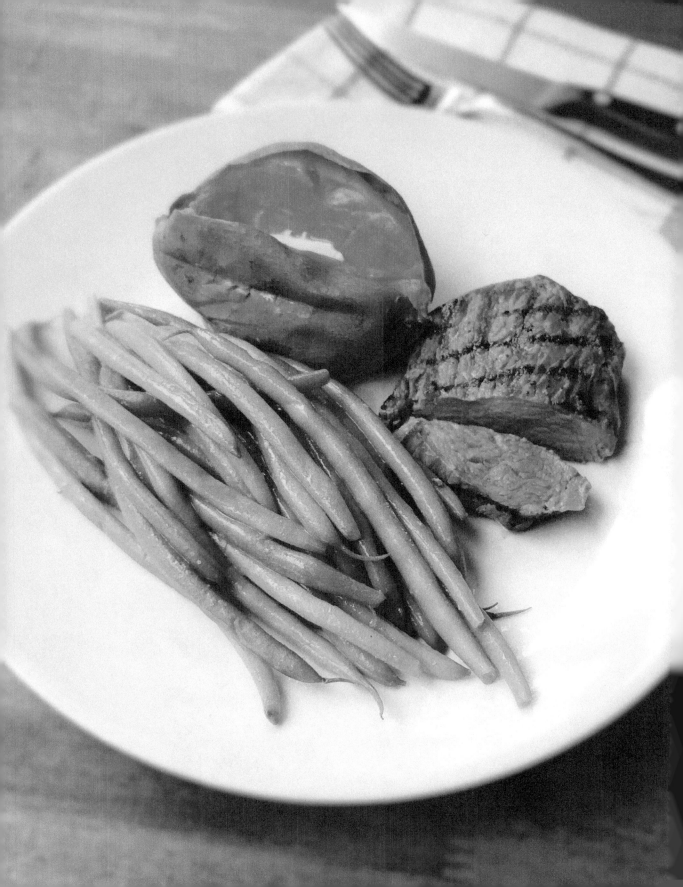

SIRLOIN STEAK WITH SWEET POTATO AND GREEN BEANS

Servings: 2* | Prep Time: 10 min | Cook Time: 45-50 min

Simple 1-2-3 Eat! for the win. If you don't have a grill or it's too cold to grill (that's hard to imagine for me), then you can use the pan/oven method. Honestly, as much as I love the grill, the other method turns out a really good steak.

*This recipe makes 2 servings of steak and one serving of everything else. Save the second serving of the steak for lunch..

8 oz sirloin steak

4 oz green beans, trimmed

1 sweet potato or yam, small

salt

pepper

butter

1. Preheat oven to 400 F. Pierce potato, and place in a baking dish (to catch the drips). Bake at 400 F for 40-55 minutes or until tender. Serve with butter, salt, and pepper if desired.

2. Preheat grill. Season steak with salt and pepper. Grill 2-4 minutes per side or until steaks have been cooked to desired doneness. (Remember they will continue to cook as they rest.) Save half of the steak for tomorrow's lunch.

3. Bring 1 quart of water to a rolling boil. Add green beans when water is fully boiling and cook for exactly 7 minutes. Drain. Serve with salt, pepper, and butter if desired.

4. PAN/OVEN METHOD: If you don't want to grill the steak, you can use a skillet and the oven. Melt some butter in an oven-proof skillet (such as a cast iron skillet) on high heat. Sear the steak in the hot butter for 2 minutes per side. Transfer the skillet to a 400 F oven for 6-8 minutes or until steaks are cooked to your liking. You may also use a regular skillet and transfer the steaks to a baking sheet.

SWEET POTATO SHEPHERD'S PIE

Servings: 2 | Prep Time: 15 min | Cook Time: 45 min

The test group was really surprised by this one. Many of them looked at this recipe with some heavy skepticism, but then they raved. I can see why. The ingredients list looks long and it's a casserole with sweet potatoes. Give it a chance and see why this became an unexpected favorite.

This recipe makes 2 servings. Save the second serving for lunch.

1 sweet potato, large

1 Tbsp unsalted butter

1/2 tsp dried rosemary

1/2 tsp dried thyme

1/2 tsp salt

1/4 tsp pepper

1/2 lb ground beef, 90% lean or leaner

1/2 onion diced

1 stalk celery, sliced

1 carrot medium, sliced

1/2 cup mushrooms, sliced

1/2 cup frozen green peas

1/2 Tbsp bottled minced garlic

3/4 cup vegetable broth

1 Tbsp tomato paste

1 Tbsp Bragg Liquid Aminos

1/2 tsp salt

1/4 tsp pepper

paprika for garnish

1. Preheat oven to 400 F.

2. Peel and dice potato. Add to a saucepan and cover with water. Bring to a boil and boil 5-7 minutes or until the diced potatoes are soft. Drain and transfer to a large bowl along with butter, rosemary, thyme, salt and pepper. Mash with an immersion blender or transfer to a food processor (or mash by hand with a fork).

3. In a skillet, brown beef and remove from pan. Set aside. NOTE: If you already cooked the beef on day 1 as suggested, this is already done but you'll need to add a little olive oil or other cooking fat for the next step since you won't have any from the beef. Just a teaspoon or so will do the trick.

4. In the same pan, cook onions, celery, carrots and mushrooms. Cook 6-8 minutes.

5. Add beef, peas, garlic, broth, paste, liquid aminos, salt, and pepper. Stir well, and bring to a boil. Reduce heat and let simmer 10-15 minutes.

6. Transfer filling to a small greased baking dish. Top with sweet potato mixture. Sprinkle with paprika. Bake at 400 for 20 minutes.

7. Serve half and save the rest of the dish for lunch.

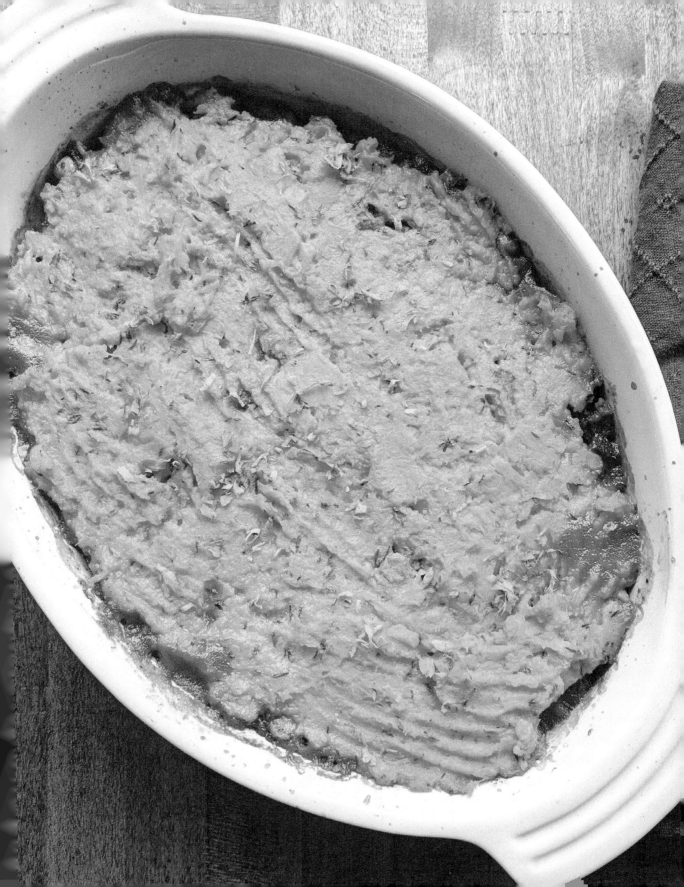

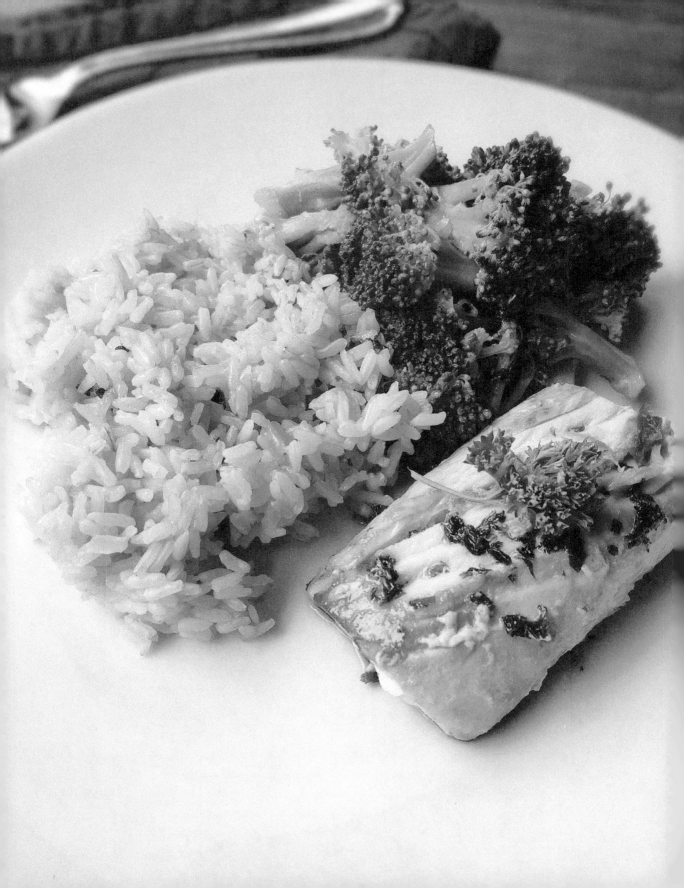

BASIL BUTTER MAHI-MAHI WITH BROWN RICE AND BROCCOLI

Servings: **2*** | Prep Time: **10 min** | Cook Time: **45-50 min**

This Mahi-Mahi is cooked in butter (grass-fed is best) and then doused in an herbed basil and parsley butter. It's paired with brown rice and simple steamed broccoli for a complete meal.

*You're making 2 servings of the fish. The second one will be used with a lunch recipe.

2 mahi-mahi fillets, 4 oz each

2 Tbsp butter, divided

1/2 Tbsp fresh basil, finely chopped

1/2 tsp fresh parsley, finely chopped

1/2 Tbsp bottled minced garlic, or fresh minced

1/4 tsp salt

1 1/2 cups broccoli florets

1/2 cup brown rice, cooked

1. Add 1/2 Tbsp of butter to a skillet and melt over medium heat.

2. Add the mahi-mahi fillets and cook approximately 4 minutes on each side until the fish is opaque. Don't overcook or it will become chewy.

3. Meanwhile, in a saucepan, melt the rest of the butter and add the fresh herbs, garlic and salt.

4. Serve by pouring the herbed butter over the fish.

5. Put about 1 inch of water into a sauce pan and add your steamer basket. Add the broccoli to the steamer basket and bring the water to a boil. Steam the broccoli over boiling water for about 4 minutes.

6. You should have brown rice from your weekly prep. If not, you can make it per the instructions on page 178.

STEAK STIR FRY WITH BROWN RICE

Servings: 2 | Prep Time: 10 min | Cook Time: 15 min

This is just a simple but colorful stir fry with cooked brown rice. You should have some brown rice from prep to make this easy. If not, you can make some per the recipe on page 178.

This recipe makes 2 servings. Save the second serving for lunch.

1 Tbsp coconut oil

1/2 lb flank steak, sliced thinly against the grain

1/2 lb sugar snap pea pods

1 carrot, large, cut into matchsticks

1/2 pint mushrooms, sliced

1 small red bell pepper, cut into thin strips

1 small zucchini, cut into thin strips

1 green onion, thinly sliced

1/2 tsp sesame seeds

1 cup brown rice, cooked (1/2 cup per serving)

Stir Fry Sauce

1 tsp cornstarch, gluten free

1 1/2 Tbsp water

1 1/2 Tbsp Bragg Liquid Aminos

1/4 inch fresh ginger, minced

1 tsp bottled minced garlic

1/4 tsp sesame oil

1. Heat coconut oil over medium high heat. Add steak. Cook, stirring frequently, 2-3 minutes. Remove from pan and keep warm.

2. In same pan, add carrots and red pepper. Stir fry 2 minutes, stirring frequently. Add mushrooms, zucchini, and peapods. Stir fry another 2-4 minutes. Return beef to pan.

3. Stir cornstarch with 1 1/2 tbsp water. Set aside.

4. Mix Bragg, ginger, garlic, and sesame oil. Pour over veggies and beef in pan, and stir in cornstarch mix. Heat, stirring constantly, until sauce thickens, about 1 minute. Remove from heat and sprinkle with green onions and sesame seeds.

5. Divide into 2 servings. Serve over cooked brown rice.

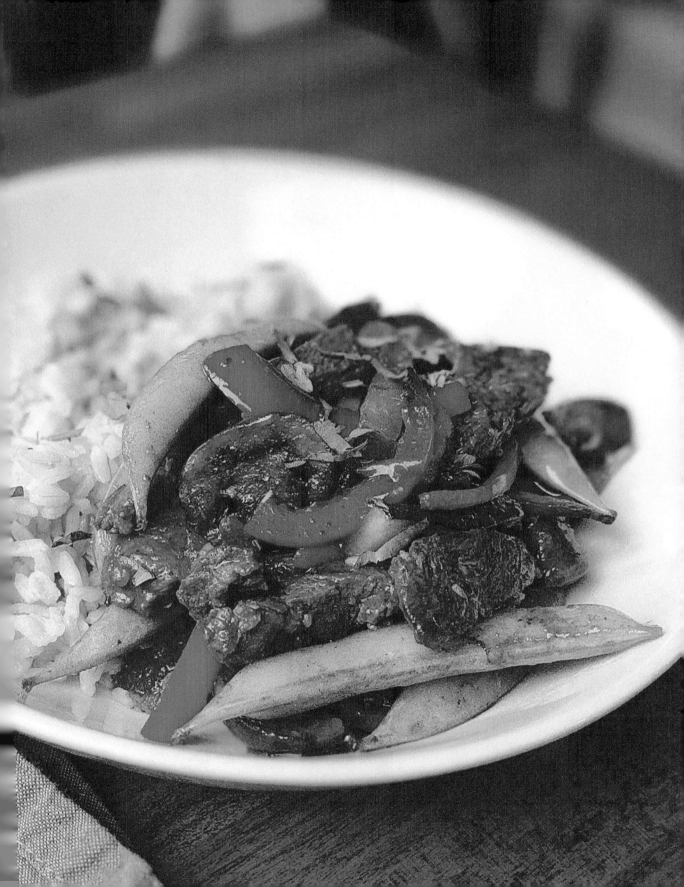

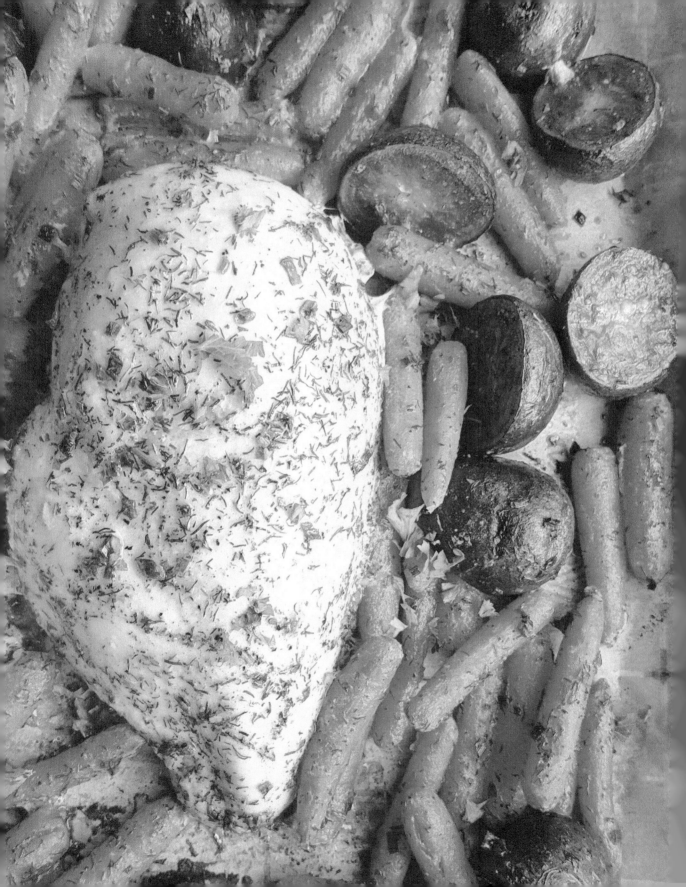

ONE PAN GARLIC RANCH CHICKEN AND VEGGIES

Servings: 2 | Prep Time: 10 min | Cook Time: 25-30 min

Another easy prep, easy clean-up sheet pan recipe!

This recipe makes 2 servings. Save the second serving for lunch.

10-12 oz boneless, skinless chicken breast (~1 large)

8 oz purple potatoes, halved

8 oz baby carrots

1 Tbsp bottled minced garlic

1 tsp salt

1/2 tsp pepper

1 Tbsp extra virgin olive oil

1/2 Tbsp onion powder

1/2 Tbsp dried chives

1/2 Tbsp dried parsley

1/2 Tbsp dried dill

1/4 cup fresh parsley, chopped, for garnish

1. Preheat oven to 400 F. Line baking sheet with parchment paper or foil.

2. Combine all ingredients except fresh parsley in a large bowl. Toss well to coat. Arrange chicken and vegetables in a single layer on prepared baking sheet.

3. Bake, uncovered, 25-30 minutes or until chicken is cooked through and vegetables are tender-crisp. Broil for 2-3 minutes, or until beginning to char. Sprinkle with fresh parsley.

4. Divide into 2 servings. Save one serving for lunch.

TERIYAKI SALMON WITH BROWN RICE AND KALE

Servings: 1 | Prep Time: 35 min* | Cook Time: 25-30 min

The flavor of this salmon is so wonderful. Salmon is great with just some lemon, but it's nice to change things up a bit sometimes.

*Note the 30 min fridge time. This is optional but recommnended.

1 salmon fillet, 6 oz each

2 Tbsp Bragg Liquid Aminos

1 tsp pure maple syrup

1/2 Tbsp bottled minced garlic

1 Tbsp lemon juice

1/2 tsp sesame oil

1/4 tsp salt

1 green onion, chopped, optional garnish

sesame seeds, optional garnish

1/2 cup brown rice, cooked

2 cups kale, destemmed and chopped

1 tsp extra virgin olive oil

1 tsp lemon juice

1. Place salmon fillet in a glass baking dish. Combine next 6 ingredients and pour over salmon. Cover and refrigerate 30 minutes.

2. Preheat grill to medium. Place salmon on grill basket or foil. Grill 2-4 minutes per side or until salmon is cooked through. Finish with chopped green onions and sesame seeds if desired. You may also cook under the broiler if you prefer (8-10 min on high depending on the thickness of your fillet).

3. You should have brown rice already cooked from prep, or you can make it from the recipe on page 178.

4. To steam the kale, place the kale in a steamer basket over boiling water for 3-5 minutes. Toss with 1 Tsp olive oil, 1 Tsp lemon juice, and salt.

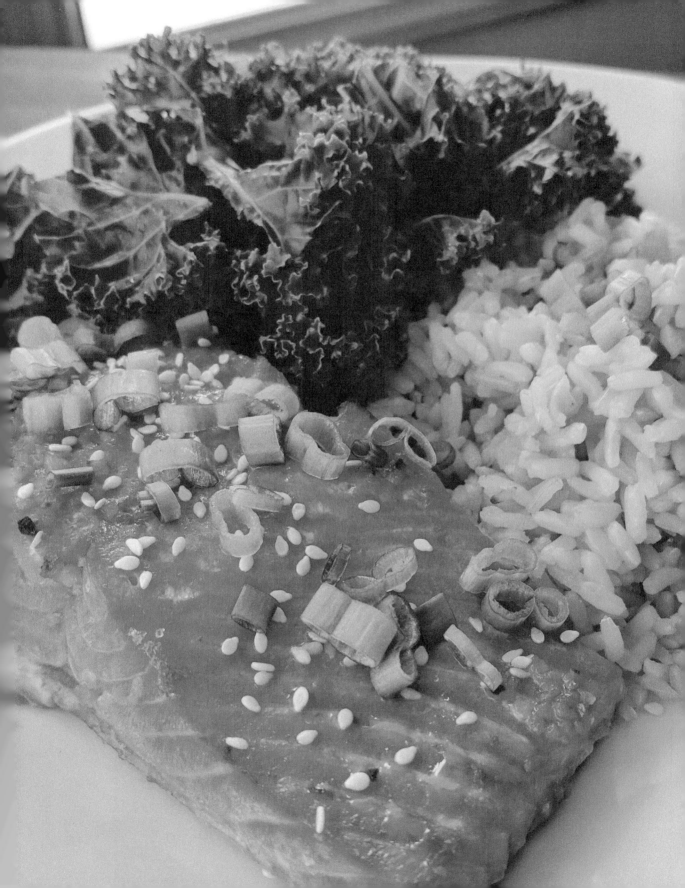

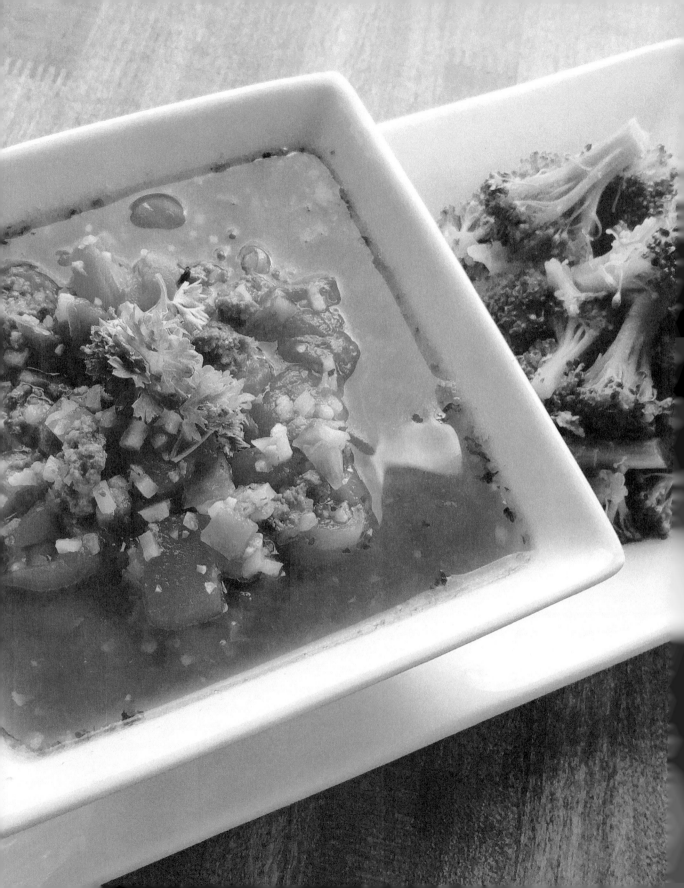

BEEF AND PEPPER SOUP WITH BROCCOLI

Servings: 2* | Prep Time: 10 min | Cook Time: Slow Cook

This recipe goes in the slow cooker and cooks all day. If you don't have a slow cooker, you can use the stove top instructions if you wish, but I like to let it cook all day.

Note that the recipe calls for 2/3 of a pound of ground beef. The other 1/3 of a pound will be used in a different recipe (don't brown it with this recipe, just save it raw in the fridge).

*Also, the soup recipe makes at least 2 servings. You'll use 1 for a lunch. You will not make 2 servings of the broccoli.

2/3 lb ground beef, 90% lean or leaner

1/2 cup frozen or fresh diced onions

1/2 cup frozen or fresh diced carrots

2/3 cup frozen bell pepper mix or 1 fresh bell pepper, diced or in strips

1/2 cup cauliflower, riced/minced

1 can crushed or petite diced tomatoes, 15 oz

1 cup beef broth

1 tsp dried basil

1 tsp oregano

1 Tbsp bottled minced garlic

salt to taste

pepper to taste

2 cups broccoli, steamed

butter, optional

1. Place all ingredients (except broccoli and butter) in a slow cooker and cook on low for 6 hours or high for 4 hours.

2. You can brown the meat first if you wish. It works either way, but some prefer to brown the meat.

3. If you don't have a slow cooker: crumble and brown the meat in a skillet. Drain. Add browned meat and all other ingredients (except broccoli and butter) in a large saucepan. Bring to a low boil over med-high heat. Reduce heat to low and simmer for 15 minutes.

4. To steam the broccoli, place in a steamer basket over boiling water for 5 minutes. Mix with butter and salt, if desired, and serve as a side to the soup.

BALSAMIC GRILLED CHICKEN AND VEGGIES

Servings: 2 | Prep Time: 20 min* | Cook Time: 25 min

This one is great on the grill, but you can make a sheet pan meal out of it if you prefer. I prefer the grill on this one, so do that if you can.

*Note the 1 hour marinating time.

This recipe makes 2 servings, so make sure to save half for lunch.

8-12 oz boneless, skinless chicken breast

1/2 red onion, cut into large chunks

1 zucchini, cut into bite sized chunks

1 yellow squash, cut into bite sized chunks

1/2 pint mushrooms, sliced or whole

1 red bell pepper, cut into large chunks

1 orange bell pepper, cut into large chunks

Marinade

1/4 cup extra virgin olive oil

1/4 cup balsamic vinegar

1 Tbsp bottled minced garlic

2 Tbsp honey

1 tsp pepper

1 tsp salt

1. Combine all vegetables and half marinade ingredients in a large zip top bag. Combine the chicken and the other half of the marinade in a second zip top bag. Toss well to coat. Let marinate 1 hour.

2. Preheat grill to medium. Add vegetables to a grill basket and chicken directly to grill. Grill 18-25 minutes (stirring vegetables regularly and turning chicken regularly) or until vegetables are tender-crisp and chicken is cooked through.

3. If you don't want to grill, you can put everything on a sheet pan in the oven at 400 F for 20 minutes or until the chicken is cooked through.

4. Save half of the recipe for lunch.

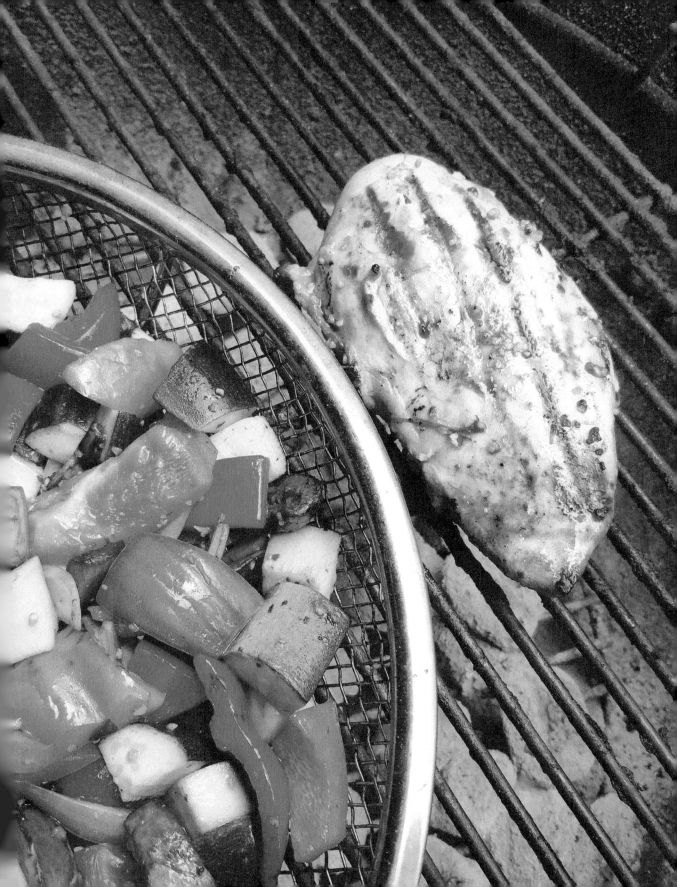

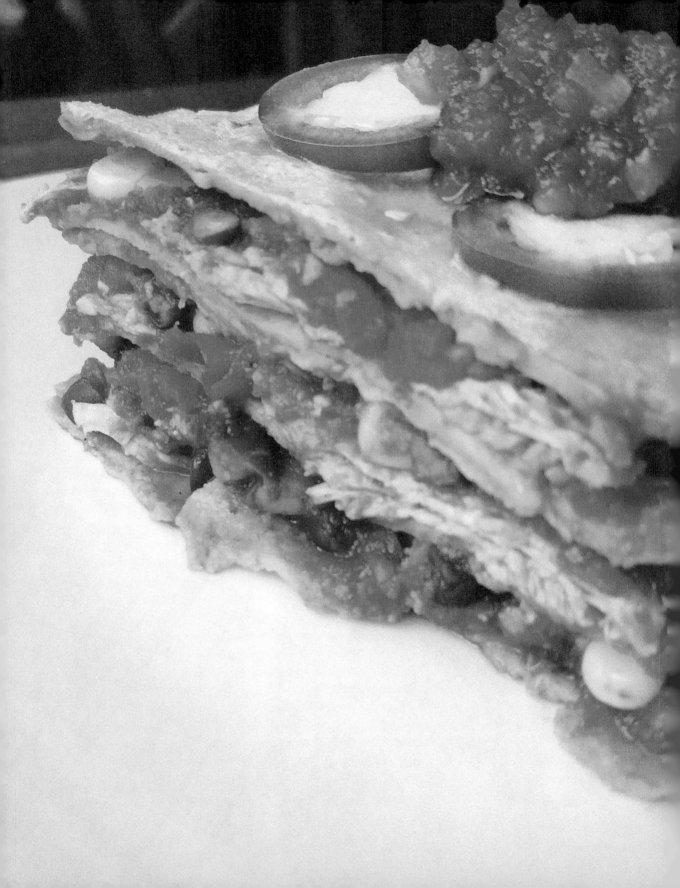

MEXICAN LASAGNA

Servings: 3 | Prep Time: 15 min | Cook Time: 30 min

Mexican lasagna is a fantastic fusion of tacos and lasagna. It's all the flavors of tasty chicken tacos in a layered casserole format.

This recipe makes 3 servings, so you have 2 servings ready for lunches for the next two days!

1 can diced tomatoes, 15 oz

1 can black beans, 15 oz, rinsed and drained

1 cup frozen corn

2 tsp chili powder

1 tsp paprika

1/4 tsp garlic powder

1/4 tsp onion powder

1/8 tsp cumin

1/8 tsp cayenne pepper

1/2 tsp salt

8 corn tortillas

1 lb boneless, skinless chicken breasts, cooked and shredded

1 cup salsa, no sugar listed in ingredients, optional

1 green onion, sliced, optional

2 oz black olives, sliced, optional

1 jalapeno, fresh sliced, optional

1. Preheat oven to 375 F.

2. You can cook the chicken just about any way you like. One of my favorites is to cover chicken breasts in water or broth in the Instant Pot and cook on high pressure for 15 minutes and then allow natural pressure release for at least 10 minutes. You can also just boil them or bake them until juices run clear.

3. Shred the chicken. If you have a Kitchen Aid mixer or even a handheld mixer, you can shred the chicken with that. In the stand mixer, it works best with the flat beater attachment (usually white and solid), but it also works with the standard beaters on a handheld mixer. You can also just shred the chicken with two forks.

4. Mix tomatoes, dry seasonings, black beans, and corn in a medium bowl. Set aside.

5. Grease an 8 x 8 casserole dish. Add a layer of corn tortillas, slightly overlapping edges. Top with 1/3 of the shredded chicken. Top with 1 cup of tomato mixture.

6. Repeat layers 3 times, or until all ingredients are used. I ended with corn tortillas on the top and I really enjoyed the crispy top layer, but you could also end with the tomato mixture.

7. Bake at 375 F for 30 minutes. Slice and serve with optional toppings.

ORANGE SALMON WITH BROWN RICE AND GREEN BEANS

Servings: 2* | Prep Time: 10 min | Cook Time: 15 min

Orange salmon is another great way to make salmon that really brings out the flavor.

*You'll make 2 servings of the salmon and use the second one in some simple lettuce wraps for lunch.

2 salmon fillets, 4-6 oz each, wild caught preferred

juice from 1 orange

1/2 tsp chili powder

1/2 tsp grated orange rind

1/4 tsp cumin

1/4 tsp paprika

1/4 tsp salt

1/8 tsp ground coriander

1/4 tsp pepper

1/2 lb green beans, fresh

butter, optional

1/2 cup brown rice, cooked

1. Preheat broiler. Mix orange juice and all remaining ingredients except green beans, butter and brown rice. Rub onto salmon.

2. Place salmon on a parchment lined baking sheet. Broil for 8 minutes or until fish is opaque and flakes easily with fork. Save one serving for later.

3. While fish is cooking, bring 2 cups of water to a boil. Add green beans and boil 7 minutes. Drain and serve with butter and salt.

4. Serve with brown rice. You should have some that you made during prep, but if not, use the recipe on page 178.

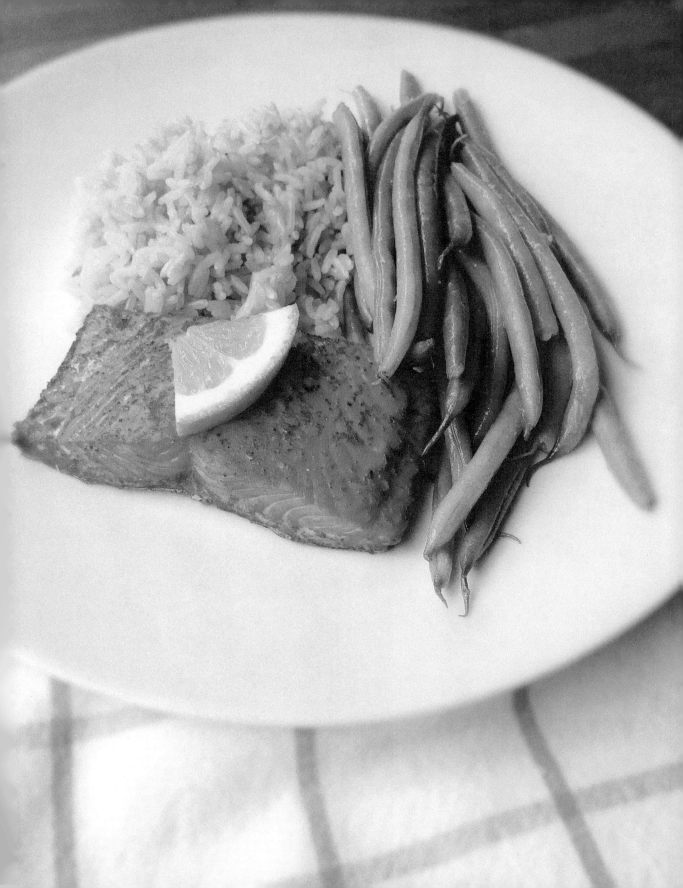

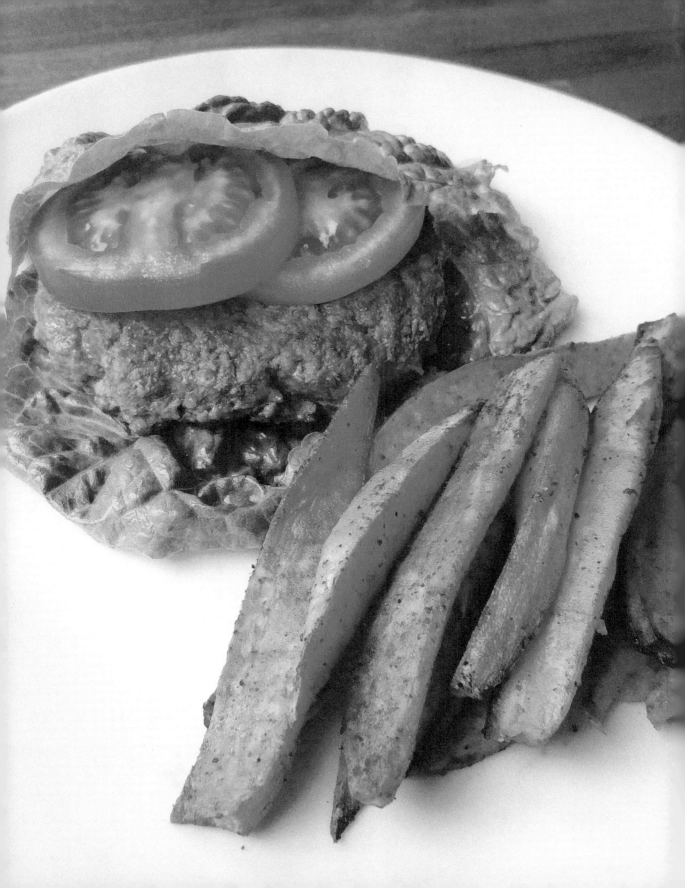

LETTUCE-WRAPPED BURGERS WITH BAKED CHILI FRIES

Servings: 1 | Prep Time: 10 min | Cook Time: 30 min

Lettuce wrapped burgers are great. Will you miss the bun? Maybe a little, but you can always add it back in after this program if you are sure you aren't sensitive to wheat.

You should have 1/3 pound of ground beef still left in the fridge for this.

3-4 oz purple or sweet potatoes

1 tsp chili powder

1 tsp extra virgin olive oil

salt

pepper

1/3 lb ground beef, 90% lean or leaner

lettuce (butter lettuce, romaine, or other green leafy lettuce)

onion, sliced

tomato, sliced

1/4 hass avocado, sliced, optional

1. Preheat oven ot 400 F. Cut the potatoes into wedges. If using sweet poatoes (as shown), peel the potatoes before cutting into wedges.

2. Combine potato wedges and olive oil in a medium bowl. Add spices. Toss to coat well.

3. Add potato wedges in a single layer on a baking sheet. Bake at 400 F for 30-40 minutes or until soft and beginning to brown. Turn broiler on and broil an additional 3 minutes.

4. While potatoes are cooking, form meat into a burger patty. Sprinkle with salt and pepper.

5. Grill or pan fry until burger has reached desired doneness.

6. Arrange patty on lettuce leaves. Top with your desired toppings. Wrap lettuce leaves around the burger. Serve with chili fries.

ONE PAN SAUSAGE AND APPLES

Servings: 2 | Prep Time: 10 min | Cook Time: 25-30 min

Sometimes uncured sausage with no sugar listed in the ingredients can be hard to find. It seems to be more common these days but if you can't find it, get the best that you can find.

You're making 2 servings with this recipe. So, be sure to make a leftover pack for lunch.

2 links uncured chicken sausage, no sugar added

1 apple, any variety

3/4 lb purple or sweet potatoes

1/2 lb baby carrots

1/2 red onion, cut into large chunks

1 Tbsp fresh sage chopped

1 Tbsp honey

2 Tbsp extra virgin olive oil

1/2 tsp salt

1/4 tsp pepper

1. Preheat the oven to 400 F. Line baking sheet with parchment paper.

2. Cut apples and onions into large chunks. Cut potatoes into smaller chunks. If you use sweet potatoes, you should also peel them.

3. Combine all ingredients in a large bowl. Toss gently to coat. Arrange on prepared baking sheet and bake for 25-35 min testing potatoes for tenderness.

4. Save half of the recipe for lunch.

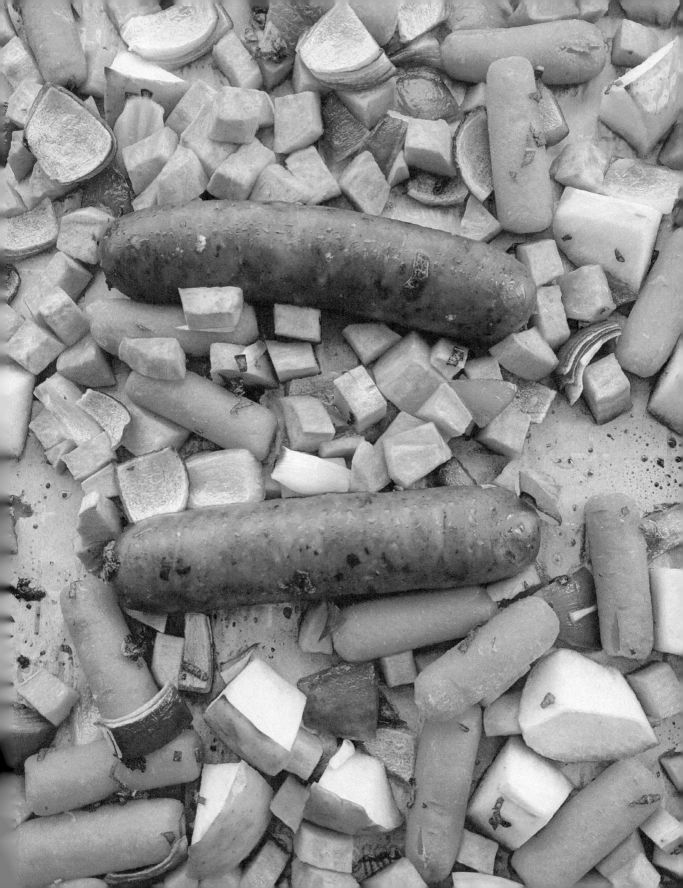

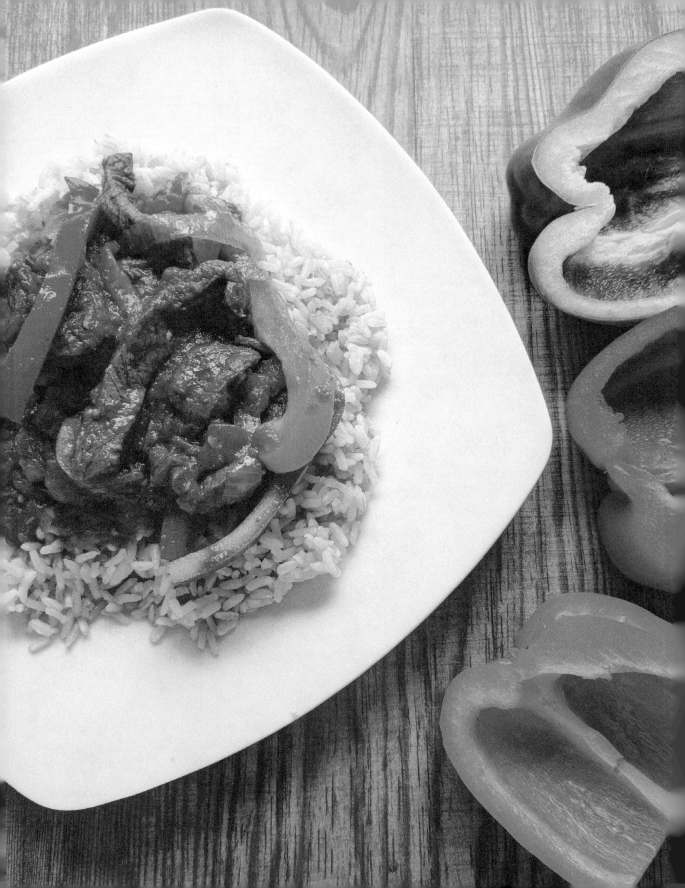

SLOW COOKER PEPPER STEAK WITH BROWN RICE

Servings: 2 | Prep Time: 10 min | Cook Time: Slow Cook

This one can just cook all day and be ready for you at dinner time. In fact, if you don't mind your peppers cooking all day, you can even add those at the beginning.

You are making 2 servings so you can start next week with a lunch ready to go.

10 oz sirloin steak, thinly sliced against the grain

1/4 tsp salt

1/4 tsp pepper

1 can crushed tomatoes, 15 oz

1/4 cup Bragg Liquid Aminos

1/3 onion, sliced or grated

1 Tbsp bottled minced garlic

1 bell pepper, seeded and sliced

1 cup brown rice, cooked

1. Add steak to slow cooker. Sprinkle with salt and pepper.

2. Add all remaining ingredients except bell peppers. Cook on low 6 hours or on high 4 hours.

3. Add peppers. Stir well. Cook an additional 60 min on high.

4. Serve over cooked brown rice. You should have some that you made during prep, but if not, use the recipe on page 178.

5. NOTE: You are welcome to add the peppers at the beginning as well. They cook down quite a bit, but they are still flavorful and wonderful. I just find that most people prefer to add them later.

PORK FRIED RICE

Servings: 3 | Prep Time: 15 min | Cook Time: 25-30 min

You can make this one in the Instant Pot or the stove top.

You're making 3 servings here so you'll have 2 lunches from this recipe as well.

2 tsp sesame oil

1/2 small onion, diced

1 large carrot, diced

1 Tbsp bottled minced garlic

1/4 inch fresh ginger, minced

1 cup brown rice, uncooked (or 2 cups cooked, see instructions)

1/4 tsp salt

1/8 tsp pepper

1 cup chicken broth or water

1/2 lb boneless pork chops

1/2 cup frozen green peas

Bragg Liquid Aminos to taste

1 green onion sliced, for garnish

1 egg

Instant Pot

1. Press "sauté" on the Instant Pot. Add the sesame oil and let it heat up. Add onion, garlic, ginger, and carrot. Sauté 3-5 min.

2. Add brown rice, salt, and pepper. Sauté for 3 minutes. Push "cancel".

3. Add chicken broth or water, mix well, and scrape bottom and edges of the insert so all of the rice and veggies are in the liquid. Dice the pork into 1/2 inch cubes and add on top of the rice mixture. Do not mix. Close the Instant Pot lid and set the valve to "sealing". Program for manual-high and 22 minutes.

4. Allow for 10 min natural pressure release, then carefully vent the rest of the pressure.Remove the lid and add the frozen peas to the rice mixture in the Instant Pot and stir well.

5. Put the lid back on the Instant Pot and move the valve to sealing. Leave sealed but not on for 5 minutes and then release pressure.

6. While the peas are steaming in the Instant Pot, beat the egg and scramble it in a skillet until it is dried out.

7. Remove the Instant Pot lid and add the eggs and mix well. Serve with Bragg liquid aminos and sliced green onions, if desired.

Stove Top

1. Cook brown rice in a rice cooker or on the stove top (see recipe on page 178 if needed).

2. Dice the pork chops into 1/2 inch cubes. Heat sesame oil in large skillet. Add pork. Cook, stirring constantly, 7 min or until cooked through. Set aside.

3. Add vegetables to skillet. Cook 2 min. Add cooked rice and ginger and sauté 2 min. Scrape veggies and rice to one side or make a well in the center. Beat the egg and pour onto the pan. Cook while stirring until scrambled.

4. Return pork to pan and stir well. Add Bragg's and sliced green onions if desired.

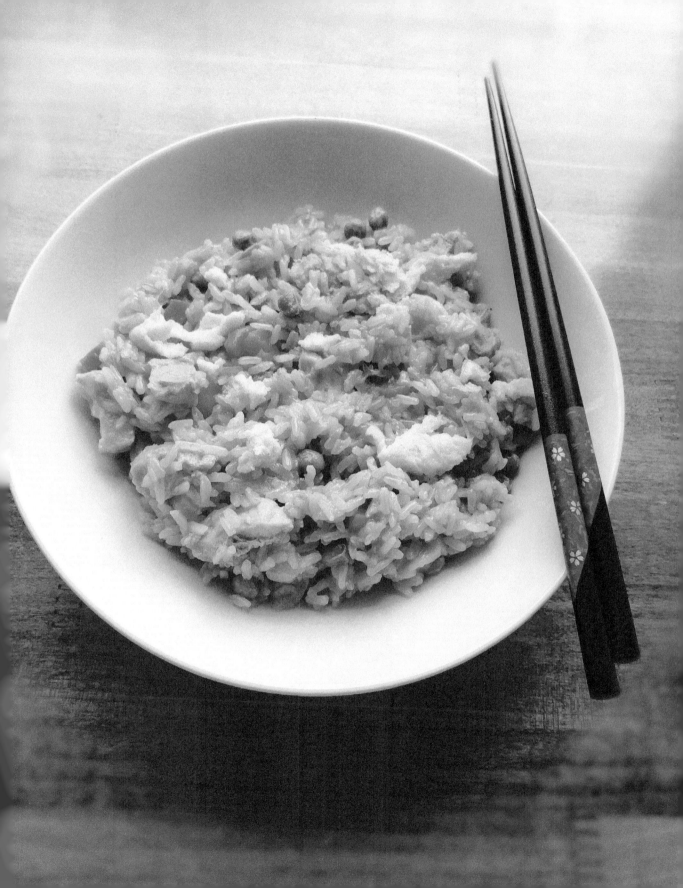

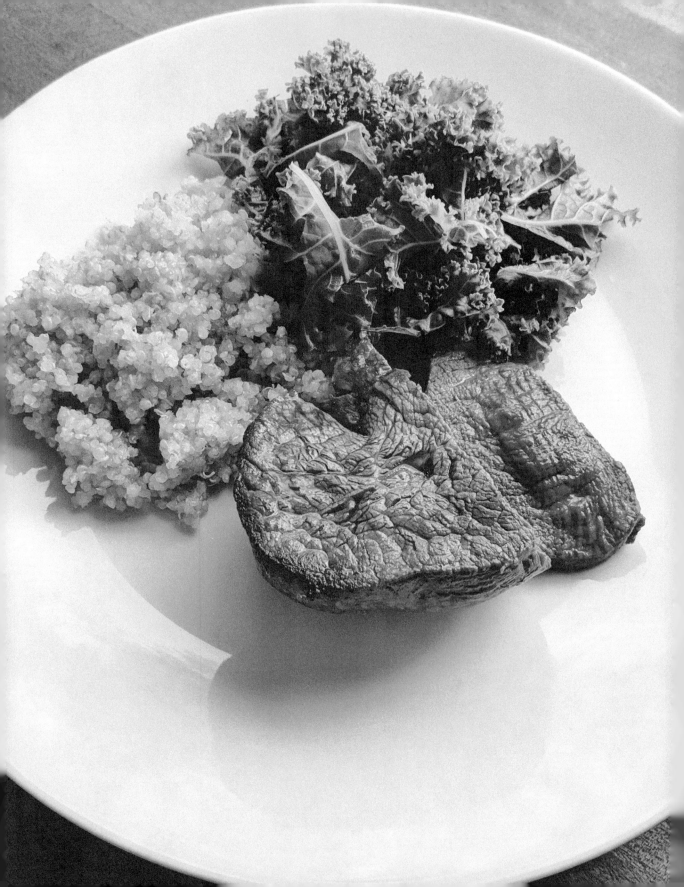

BUTTER PAN STEAK WITH STEAMED KALE AND QUINOA

Servings: 2* | Prep Time: 10 min | Cook Time: 25 min

If you've never cooked steak this way, you're in for a treat! The idea here is to get a good "crust" on the steak in the first part and then finish the inside in the oven. It comes out fantastic.

*You are making 2 servings of the steak to use as a salad topping, but you won't make 2 servings of the sides.

8 oz sirloin steak, grass-fed if possible

salt

pepper

1/4 cup quinoa, uncooked

1/2 cup water

1 1/2 Tbsp butter, grass-fed if possible

3 cups kale, destemmed and chopped

1 Tbsp lemon juice

1 tsp extra virgin olive oil

1. Salt and pepper the steak liberally and then bring to room temperature on the counter. Preheat oven to 425 F.

2. Bring quinoa and water to a boil. Cover, reduce heat, and simmer 15 minutes or until quinoa is cooked and water is absorbed.

3. While quinoa is cooking, heat a cast iron or other oven-safe skillet to high heat on the stove and melt 1 tbsp of butter.

4. Add the steak to the pan and sear for 2 minutes on each side. You don't need to do anything for those 2 minutes but you can spoon the butter up over the top if there is room to do so in the pan.

5. Move the pan to the preheated oven and allow to cook for 6 minutes at 425 F for a 1 1/2 inch thick steak. If you're steaks are thicker, you may need slightly longer or slightly less if they are thinner. You can check with a thermometer to get the temperature you want but 6 minutes is just about right. For medium rare, if you're checking with a thermometer, remove at 140 F. The meat will continue to cook during the rest period.

6. Let the steak rest on a plate for about 5 minutes to finish cooking.

7. To steam the kale, place the kale in a steamer basket over boiling water for 3-5 minutes (covered). Toss with 1 Tbsp olive oil, 1 Tbsp lemon juice, and salt.

8. Save half of the steak for lunch.

WHITE CHICKEN CHILI

Servings: 2 | Prep Time: 10 min | Cook Time: Slow Cook

White chicken chili is quite a bit different than the chili you had earlier in this plan. It's just as easy to make, but gives you unique flavor with green chiles and chicken.

This recipe makes 2 servings, so you'll have one for a lunch later in the week.

1 lb boneless, skinless chicken breasts

1 Tbsp bottled minced garlic

1 can green chiles, 4 oz

1 Tbsp cumin

1/2 tsp oregano

1/4 tsp cayenne pepper, optional

1 1/2 cups chicken broth

1 can white beans, 15 oz, drained and rinsed

1 green bell pepper, diced

cilantro, fresh chopped, optional

1. Combine all ingredients except cilantro in a slow cooker.

2. Cook on high 4 hours or low for 6 hours. Shred chicken with 2 forks. Top with cilantro if desired.

3. If you don't have a slow cooker, just cook the chicken first by dicing it and sautéing it in a little olive oil until juices run clear. Then add everything except cilantro to a large saucepan and heat over medium heat for about 30 minutes to warm through and let flavors meld.

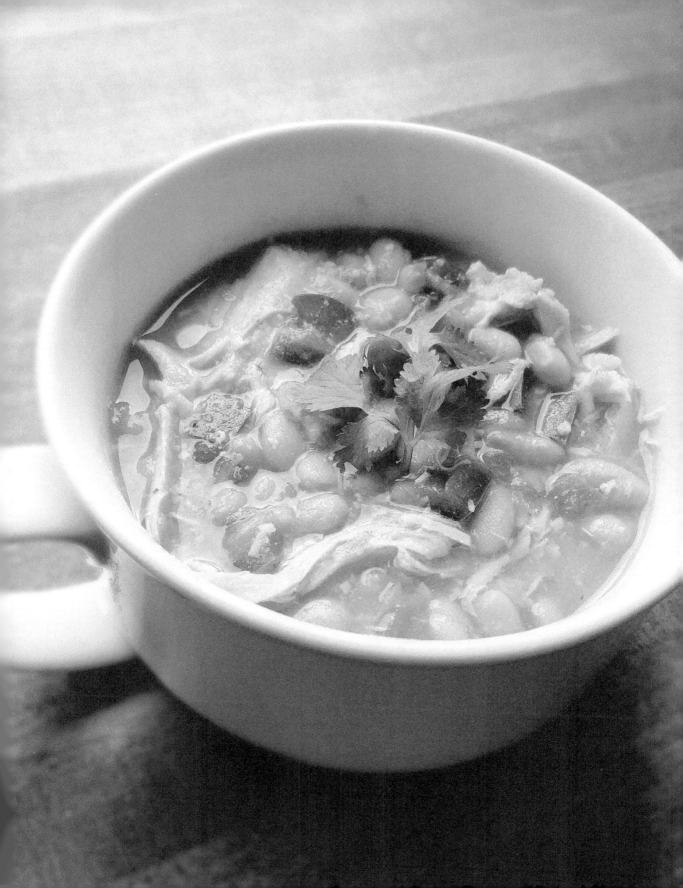

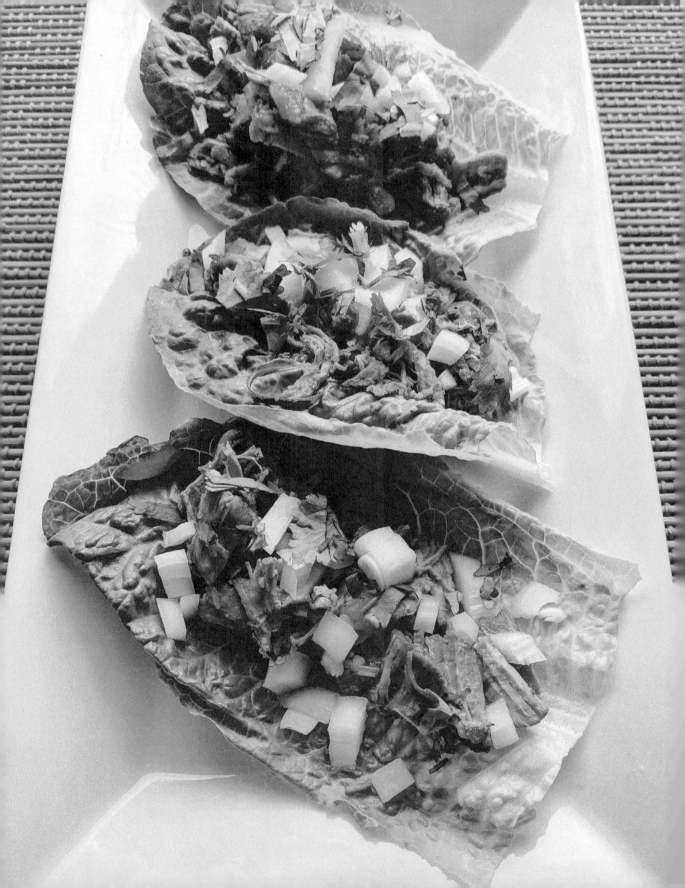

LETTUCE-WRAPPED PORK CARNITAS TACOS

Servings: 2* | Prep Time: 10 min | Cook Time: Slow Cook

Tacos! Did I mention that I love Mexican yet? Maybe once. Just wrap up the carnitas in the lettuce and add some onions and cilantro.

NOTE: It's pretty hard to find a ¾ lb pork tenderloin. So, the plan is to buy 1.5 pounds and use half here and the other half for the pork and veggies later this week. Perfect. *You'll save half of this meat for a salad topping.

3/4 lb of pork tenderloin

1/2 Tbsp chipotle chile powder

1 tsp cumin

1/2 tsp pepper

1/2 tsp chili powder

2 tsp salt

1 Tbsp extra virgin olive oil optional, for searing

1 cup chicken broth

1 onion, medium, diced (divided)

1 Tbsp bottled minced garlic

3-4 large lettuce leaves such as romaine or butter lettuce

cilantro, fresh, chopped

1. Cut the pork into large slices (about 3/4" thick).

2. Mix the next 5 ingredients and sprinkle onto the pork. Heat oil in a large nonstick skillet. Add pork slices and sear on all sides.

3. Add pork to slow cooker along with broth, ½ of the diced onions (use the rest for topping), and garlic. Cook on low 6 hours or on high 4 hours.

4. Preheat broiler to high. Line rimmed baking sheet with foil. While broiler is preheating, shred meat with two forks. Transfer meat to baking sheet. Arrange the meat in an even layer on the baking sheet. Reserve juices.

5. Broil meat for about 5 minutes, or until the edges of the pork begin to brown and turn crispy. Remove the sheet pan from the oven and ladle about 1/4 cup of the juices over the pork. Toss to coat. Broil for an additional 5 minutes. Remove pan and ladle an additional 1/4 cup juices over meat.

6. Wrap in lettuce with fresh chopped onions and cilantro.

7. Save half of the meat for a salad topping.

THAI CHICKEN SOUP

Servings: 2 | Prep Time: 10 min | Cook Time: 15 min

This one is really quick to put together and has a wonderful coconut flavor.

This recipe makes 2 servings, so you'll have one for a lunch later in the week.

1 can coconut milk, full fat, not lite

1/2 cup chicken broth

2 tsp red curry paste

1/2 tsp salt

1/2 tsp pepper

8 oz boneless, skinless chicken breast, very thinly sliced

3 oz snow peas

1 cup bean sprouts

cilantro, fresh chopped

1. Add coconut milk, chicken broth, curry paste, salt, and pepper to a saucepan. Bring to a boil.

2. Add chicken breasts. Boil 3 minutes. Add peas and sprouts. Boil 5 minutes longer or until chicken is cooked through.

3. Top with cilantro.

4. Save half of the soup for lunch.

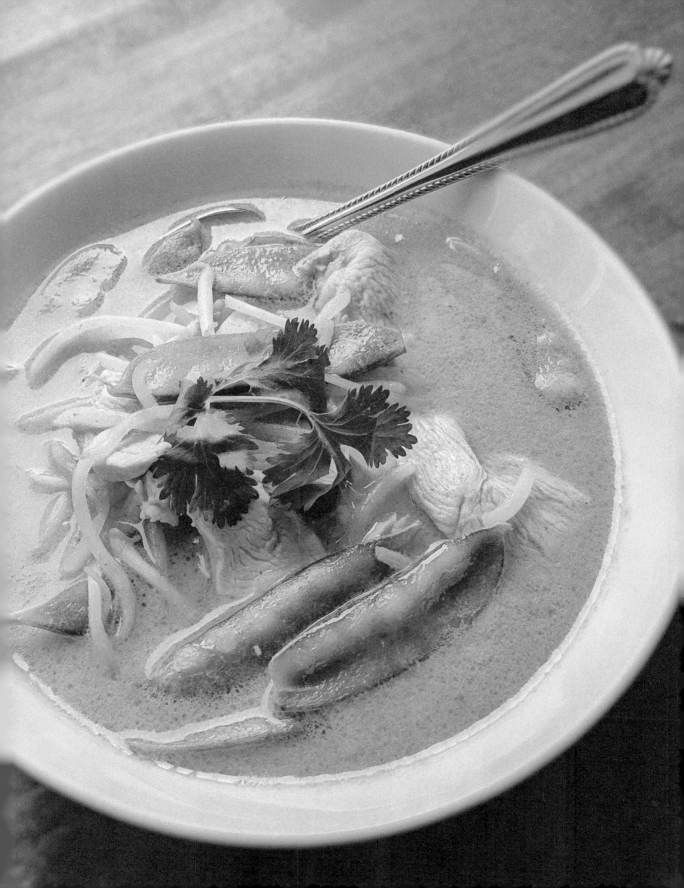

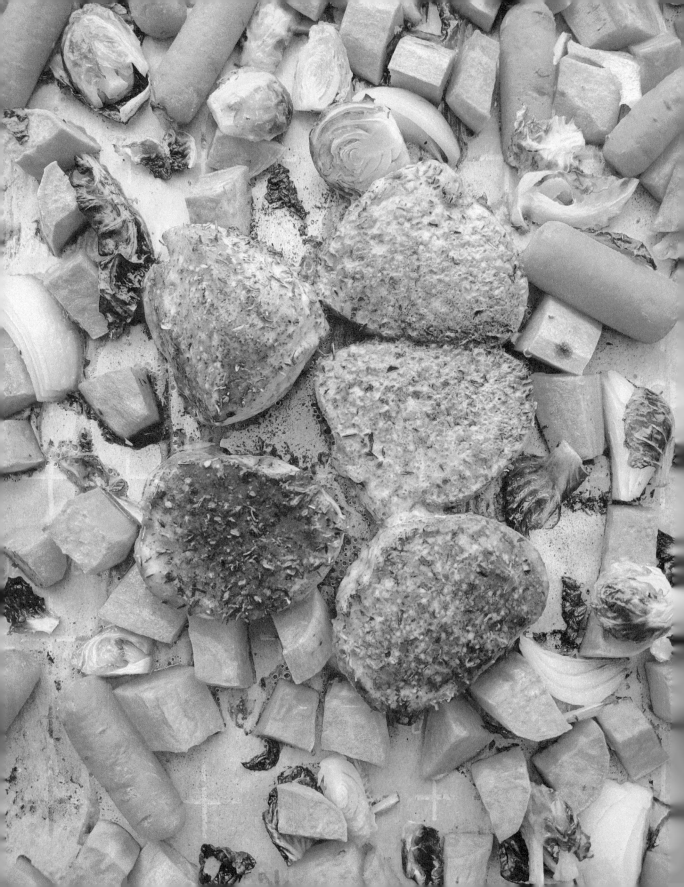

ONE PAN PORK AND VEGGIES

Servings: 2 | Prep Time: 10 min | Cook Time: 20 min

One pan for the win! You're using up the remaining pork for this week in this recipe. This will leave you with some leftovers for tomorrow as well (even though the program is technically over).

3/4 lb pork tenderloin

1 tsp paprika

1 tsp oregano

1 tsp dried thyme

1/2 tsp salt

1/2 tsp pepper

6 oz Brussels sprouts, stemmed and halved

4 oz baby carrots

3/4 lbs sweet potatoes, peeled and cut into 1 inch chunks

1/2 onion cut into wedges

1 1/2 Tbsp extra virgin olive oil

1. Preheat oven to 400 F. Line a rimmed baking sheet with parchment paper or foil.

2. Cut the pork into thick slices (about 3/4 inch thick).

3. Combine all dry spices except salt and sprinkle onto the pork. Place pork in center of prepared pan.

4. Combine vegetables and oil in a medium bowl. Toss to coat. Arrange vegetables around pork.

5. Roast, uncovered, 20 minutes or until the pork juices run clear and the internal temperature of the pork reads 145 degrees. Sprinkle vegetables with salt and pepper, to taste.

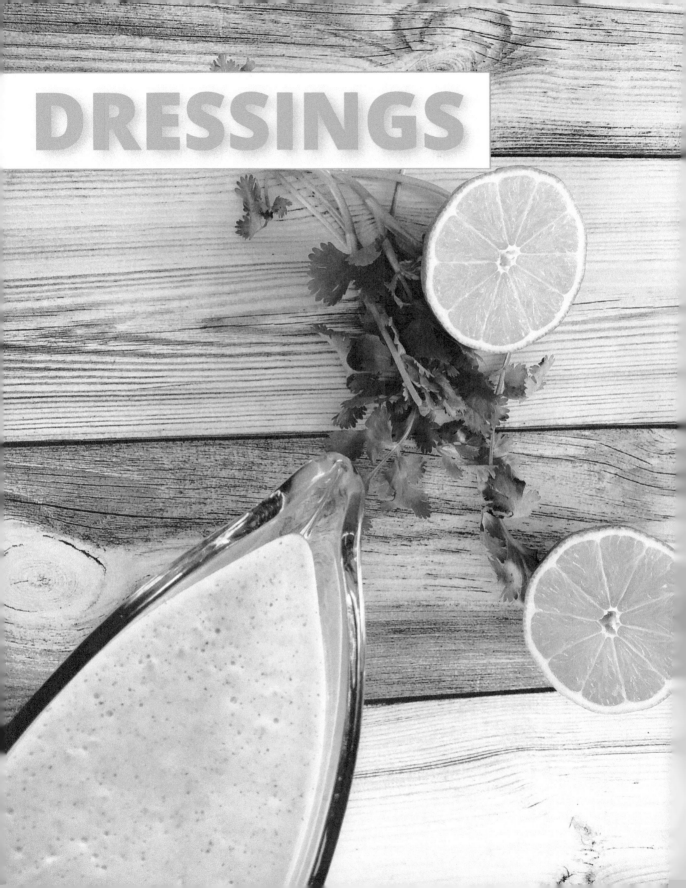

DRESSINGS

Dressings you find in the grocery store always seem to have sugar and processed junk. Although a few companies have started producing clean dressings, it can still be difficult to find healthy options. This section provides you with a variety of dressing options you can easily make during your prep time and have ready for the week. On the last page, there are also some options for commercial dressings and easy dressing ideas that don't need a recipe.

THAI PEANUT DRESSING

Servings: ~6 | Prep Time: 5 min | Cook Time: N/A

1/2 cup natural peanut butter, creamy

1/4 cup rice vinegar

1/4 cup Bragg Liquid Aminos or coconut aminos

1 Tbsp honey

2 tsp toasted sesame oil

1/4 tsp red chili flakes more or less to taste

1/4 tsp dried ginger or fresh minced

1 tsp bottled minced garlic or 1 clove fresh

1. Whisk together or combine in a blender. Store in the refrigerator for up to 1 week.

MISO GINGER DRESSING

Servings: ~6| Prep Time: 5 min | Cook Time: N/A

1/2 cup extra virgin olive oil

1/4 cup apple cider vinegar

1/4 cup miso paste, any color, no msg

2 tsp minced ginger, fresh or bottled

1 Tbsp Bragg Liquid Aminos or coconut aminos

1. Whisk together or combine in a blender. Store in the refrigerator for up to 1 week.

CREAMY GARLIC DRESSING

Servings: ~6 | Prep Time: 5 min | Cook Time: N/A

1/4 cup extra virgin olive oil

1/2 cup apple cider vinegar

1 Tbsp bottled minced garlic

3 Tbsp lemon juice

2 Tbsp fresh basil

1 tsp salt

1 Tbsp honey

1. Whisk together or combine in a blender. Store in the refrigerator for up to 1 week.

MAPLE SOY DRESSING

Servings: ~6 | Prep Time: 5 min | Cook Time: N/A

1/4 cup extra virgin olive oil

3 Tbsp sesame oil

1/2 tsp crushed red pepper

3 Tbsp pure maple syrup

2 Tbsp Bragg Liquid Aminos or coconut aminos

1. Whisk together or combine in a blender. Store in the refrigerator for up to 1 week.

CILANTRO LIME DRESSING

Servings: ~6 | Prep Time: 5 min | Cook Time: N/A

1 cup cilantro, loosely packed, stems removed

1/2 cup plain Greek yogurt

1 tsp bottled minced garlic

juice of 1 lime

1/4 cup extra virgin olive oil

2 Tbsp apple cider vinegar

1. Combine ingredients in a food processor or blender. Store in the refrigerator for up to 1 week.

HUMMUS DIP

Servings: ~5 | Prep Time: 5 min | Cook Time: N/A

1/4 cup tahini

1/4 cup lemon juice

2 Tbsp extra virgin olive oil

2 Tbsp bottled minced garlic

1 can garbanzo beans, 15 oz

1 tsp salt

1. Rinse and drain the beans. Combine ingredients in a food processor or blender. Store in the refrigerator for up to 1 week.

OTHER DRESSING OPTIONS

Olive oil and vinegar

A simple drizzle of olive oil and balsamic vinegar can be fabulous on salads and it takes no time at all.

Commercial dressings

Primal Kitchen brand makes completely green tier dressings at the time of this writing. You can find links to Thrive Market on the resources page at 28daystoclean.com/resources or use one of the QR codes found throughout this book to get there. By the time you read this, there may be a few other brands out there with green tier dressings, but you'll need to read ingredients to be sure.

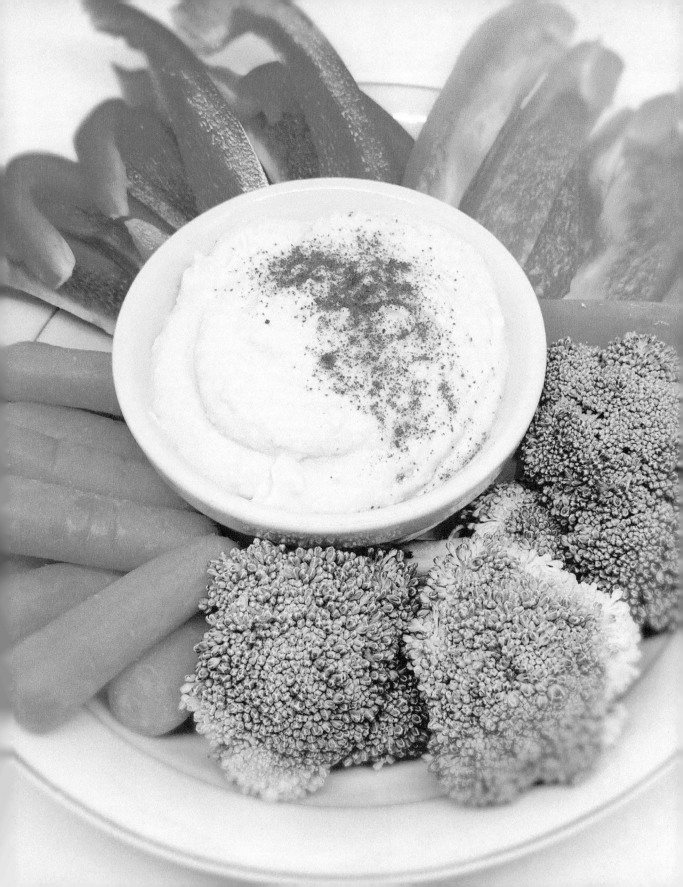

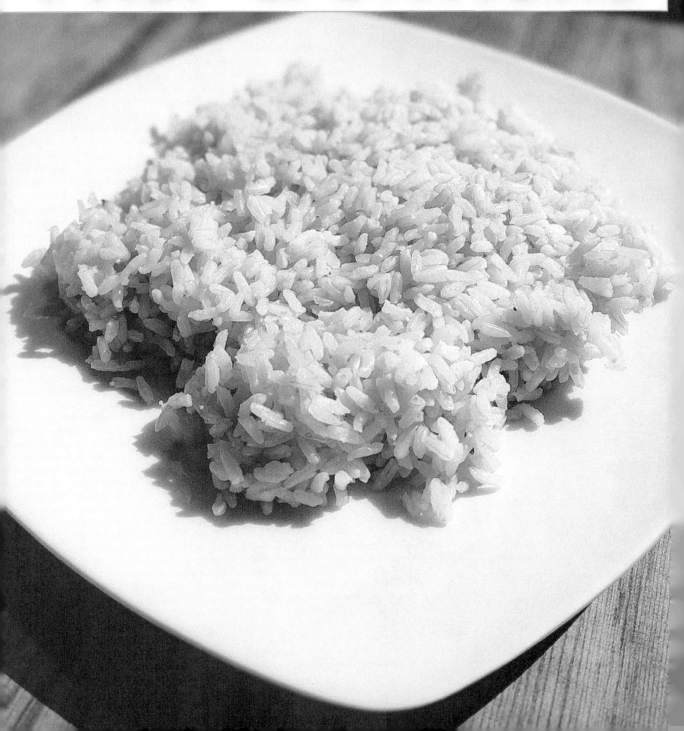

This section has a few recipes you'll use in your weekly prep as well as the list of snack options. The snack list is only limited to these options to prevent decision overload. I suggest you stick to it for the program even though there are more options available that would fit the program.

BROWN RICE

Servings: Varies | Prep Time: 5 min | Cook Time: 20-25 min

You'll need brown rice throughout the program. Often, you'll be making it during the prep for the coming week, so see the prep pages for the amounts you need for that week.

brown rice, uncooked (amount varies per week)

water (amount varies per week)

Stove Top

1. Combine uncooked brown rice and twice as much water in a saucepan (i.e. 2 cups of water for every 1 cup of uncooked brown rice). Bring to a boil.

2. Cover, reduce heat, and simmer 20 minutes or until liquid is absorbed. Fluff with fork.

3. For sticky rice, soak rice for 15 minutes prior to cooking and increase simmer time to 40 minutes.

Instant Pot

1. For the Instant Pot, use equal parts water and rice (i.e. 1 cup of water for every 1 cup of uncooked brown rice).

2. Add rice and water to the Instant Pot insert. Close lid, set to sealing, press manual (high), and set to 22 minutes.

3. For sticky rice, use a little more water than rice (1 1/4 cups water to 1 cup rice).

Rice Cooker

1. Rice cookers vary. Please follow the instructions for brown rice for your particular rice cooker.

HARD-BOILED EGGS

Servings: **Varies** | Prep Time: **< 5 min** | Cook Time: **5-10 min**

You'll need hard-boiled eggs for snacks (optional) and with some salads throughout the program. This is something that will be called out during prep for each week but it doesn't take long, so it can be made any time.

eggs (amount varies per week)

Stove Top

1. Place eggs in a saucepan. Cover them with cool water by 1 inch. Bring water to a boil over medium heat.

2. When the water is boiling, cover and remove from heat.

3. Let them stand for 10-12 minutes to cool.

4. Place the eggs in a bowl of cold water for 5 minutes. Peel and enjoy.

Instant Pot

1. Add 1 cup of water to the insert of your Instant Pot. Add the steaming rack. Add eggs on top of the rack. The eggs shouldn't be touching the water.

2. Close lid, set to sealing, press manual (high), and set to 5 minutes.

3. When the Instant Pot beeps indicating that the 5 minutes is over, let the pressure release naturally for 5 minutes and then release the rest manually. Remove lid.

4. Finally, add the eggs to a bowl of cold water for 5 minutes. When the 5 minutes is up, enjoy the easiest peeling hard-boiled eggs ever.

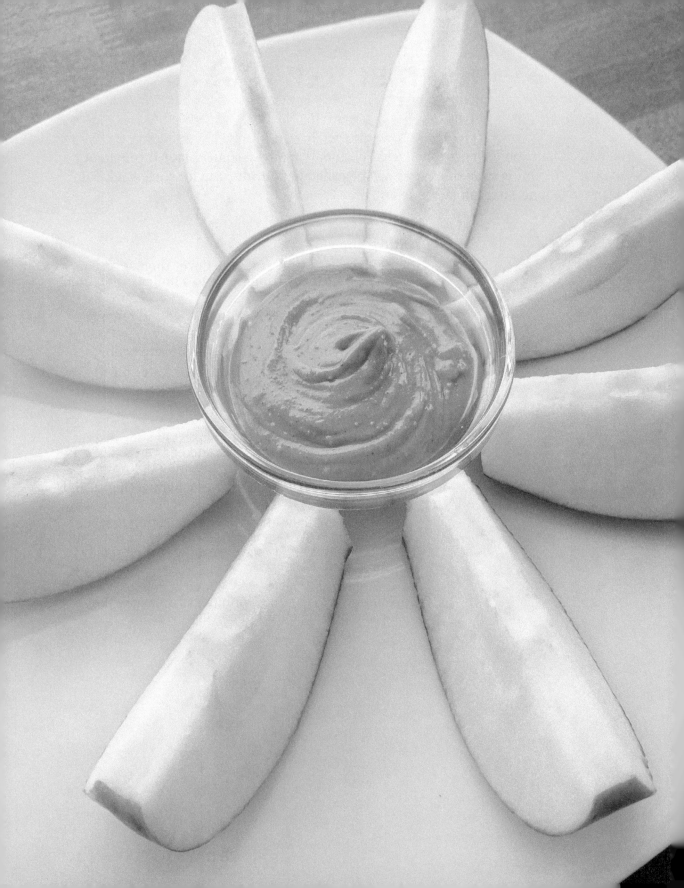

SNACK OPTIONS

There are certainly many more snack options that are green tier and healthy. However, to keep it simple, I've given you a short list to work with. If you feel comfortable picking things from the green tier to snack on, please feel free to do that. Just remember to stay away from wheat and dairy. Also, try to think about the other things you eat that day and go for diversity. If you're having the berry crisp that day, then the yogurt snack listed below isn't a good choice because you've already had yogurt with the crisp.

1 small apple, 2 Tbsp natural peanut butter or almond butter

Make sure you choose nut butter like Adam's brand that only contains peanuts and salt. If you like larger apple varieties such as Honeycrisp apples, consider only doing 1/2 of an apple

1 cup berries, 1/4 cup of almonds

You may also choose cashews, walnuts, or other nuts. Raw is best but dry roasted is fine too.

1 cup of carrots, 1/4 cup of hummus

You can often find store-bought hummus that is all green tier. If not, you can always make your own with the recipe on page 174.

Celery, 2 Tbsp natural peanut butter or almond butter

Use as much celery as you like. Make sure you choose nut butter like Adam's brand that only contains peanuts and salt.

2 hard-boiled eggs

Hard-boiled eggs make a great snack. Use the recipe on page 179.

1/2 of an avocado

Feel free to use some hot sauce or lemon juice on the avocado. This is one of my personal favorite snacks.

1 cup yogurt, 1/2 cup berries, and a drizzle of honey

Use Greek or regular yogurt (plain, unsweetened), and add fresh berries and a small drizzle of honey.

REFERENCES

Kellogg's® Smart Start® Strong Heart Antioxidants cereal smart label ingredients section, accessed on 6/13/19, <http://smartlabel.kelloggs.com/Product/Index/00038000663307#ingredients>

Walmart.com listing of Nabisco Wheat Thins Original Crackers (now discontinued and replaced with a 100% whole grain version), accessed on 6/13/19, <https://www.walmart.com/ip/Nabisco-Wheat-Thins-Original-Crackers-10-0-OZ/10292628>

Lean Cuisine Chicken Fettucine product information page, accessed on 6/13/19, <https://www.leancuisine.com/products/details/10603>

INDEX